Health Informatics

Gondy Leroy

Kathryn J. Hannah • Marion J. Ball
(Series Editors)

Designing User Studies in Informatics

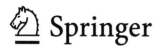 Springer

Author
Gondy Leroy Ph.D.
School of Information Systems
and Technology
Claremont Graduate University
130 E. Ninth Street
Claremont, CA 91711
USA
Gondy.Leroy@cgu.edu

ISBN 978-0-85729-621-4   e-ISBN 978-0-85729-622-1
DOI 10.1007/978-0-85729-622-1
Springer London Dordrecht Heidelberg New York

British Library Cataloguing in Publication Data
A catalogue record for this book is available from the British Library

Library of Congress Control Number: 2011934622

Cover design: eStudioCalamar, Figueres/Berlin

Printed on acid-free paper

Springer is part of Springer Science+Business Media (www.springer.com)

Health Informatics Series Preface

This series is directed to healthcare professionals leading the transformation of healthcare by using information and knowledge. For over 20 years, Health Informatics has offered a broad range of titles: some address specific professions such as nursing, medicine, and health administration; others cover special areas of practice such as trauma and radiology; still other books in the series focus on inter-disciplinary issues, such as the computer based patient record, electronic health records, and networked healthcare systems. Editors and authors, eminent experts in their fields, offer their accounts of innovations in health informatics. Increasingly, these accounts go beyond hardware and software to address the role of information in influencing the transformation of healthcare delivery systems around the world. The series also increasingly focuses on the users of the information and systems: the organizational, behavioral, and societal changes that accompany the diffusion of information technology in health services environments.

Developments in healthcare delivery are constant; in recent years, bioinformatics has emerged as a new field in health informatics to support emerging and ongoing developments in molecular biology. At the same time, further evolution of the field of health informatics is reflected in the introduction of concepts at the macro or health systems delivery level with major national initiatives related to electronic health records (EHR), data standards, and public health informatics.

These changes will continue to shape health services in the twenty-first century. By making full and creative use of the technology to tame data and to transform information, Health Informatics will foster the development and use of new knowledge in healthcare.

Preface

Informatics and Medicine

Over the last few decades informatics has played an increasingly important role in all aspects of our lives, particularly in medicine and biology. Information systems for healthcare, medicine and biology are becoming increasingly numerous and better, more fine-tuned but also more complex to develop, evaluate and use. They are being developed for a variety of reasons ranging from team decision making, improving diagnoses, educating patients and training clinicians to facilitating discovery and improving workflow. Developing good and useful systems is not simply a matter of writing efficient code. Having an information system that functions correctly and efficiently is just the beginning. Today's systems have to fit in with or improve existing conditions. They need to take strengths and weaknesses of intended users into account together with their preferences, environment, work styles and even personal characteristics. System development and implementation in any healthcare setting is further complicated by the need to focus on safety and privacy. Frequent evaluations help improve the systems by uncovering problems and providing guidance. But it's not an easy task.

Evaluating information systems and user testing fits in well with modern software development cycles. The best systems will have included evaluation by representative users from the very first development of components and will continue the interaction until the entire system has been integrated into its intended settings. The studies themselves are straightforward; deception is seldom required, there are many willing and interested stakeholders and the studies have potential to, indirectly, help improve our quality of life. However, conducting studies is often time consuming, sometimes expensive and only rewarding when the study was well enough designed so that the conclusions are valid. As a result, it is important not to waste time, money and other resources on poorly designed studies.

This book aims to be a practical guide to conducting user studies, also called controlled experiments or randomized trials. Such studies allow the experimenter to draw causal conclusions. This book focuses on designing *user* studies to test *information technology*. It is about information technology to be used by people; therefore the technology should be evaluated by people. This book will not discuss evaluations that do not include humans. For example, a database stored procedure that is being stress-tested for access and speed does not require a user study. However, studies are not limited to the evaluation of entire systems. Individual algorithms and interfaces that affect or present human interaction with a system can be evaluated separately. It is wise to test individual components when possible and not to wait until all components have been built and integrated. Early evaluations will ensure better systems and will further make the evaluation process manageable and efficient. The goal, after all, is to develop information technology that is useful and wanted, and that achieves its goal in a user-friendly, effective and efficient manner.

Currently, few books exist that are written specifically for user studies in informatics. The existing books generally belong to one of two categories. One category focuses on design and development of software in computer science and how to program, use data structures and algorithms, and design and develop complete systems. These books seldom cover user studies. As a result, many information and computer science professionals are never taught the basics of user studies. The other category of books belongs to the behavioral sciences. These books focus on measuring psychological traits, intentions and beliefs. The studies are used to build, support or refute theories and sometimes require deceiving participants. They generally require more complicated designs and associated statistical analyses than what is needed for evaluation in informatics.

This book was written to bridge the gap between informatics and the behavioral sciences. It links the two fields and combines the necessary elements from both informatics and the behavioral sciences. The most commonly used and required studies that are useful in computing are explained in detail. An overview and additional references are provided for readers who want to complement their user studies with other forms of evaluations such as case studies, quasi-experiments, or correlation studies. However, these are not the focus of this book. The included topics will provide the necessary foundation and knowledge for the majority of user studies in informatics.

The principles discussed in this book apply to all domains where information systems are employed. The examples are chosen to demonstrate individual features of evaluations. They are taken from medicine, biomedicine, biology and other healthcare-related fields. These fields were chosen because they have a high impact on our life and are incorporating technology at a fast pace. Furthermore, these fields place a strong emphasis on doing controlled studies, the randomized controlled trials that allow causal conclusions. Those are the types of studies addressed in this book. Even though there are many other types of studies that provide high quality and valuable information, randomized controlled trials are considered the gold standard in medicine and it is crucial to have a clear understanding of how to conduct them. Statistical details are included as necessary to demonstrate the underlying principles. For interested readers, references are provided to in-depth materials that served as the basis for these discussions. Since statistical software packages change and improve over time, no detailed step-by-step instructions are included. However, since the statistical models covered in this book are standard, not esoteric, pointers to commonly found options in the statistical packages, e.g., Model I or Model II specification, are included and explained.

Audience

This book is intended for managers and developers in industry and academic settings. User studies will improve software design and can demonstrate superiority. A well designed study is the cornerstone for developers to learn about the strengths and weaknesses of their algorithms and systems. This in turn leads to better products and sales, enhancing the reputation of any business. Developing information systems is very costly. By doing studies early on, the researcher and developer can increase chances of success significantly. Developing a system without errors, that provides a clear advantage and leads to high user satisfaction, is essential to any software company. Indirectly, a valid evaluation is also an excellent marketing tool for businesses. For developers in a research setting, a well designed study is necessary to get the results published at a conference or in a journal. It is also essential to winning research grant proposals.

This book is also intended for instructors and students in the different flavors of the informatics fields. Over the years, there has been little focus on conducting user studies in most computing majors. This trend has significant consequences. At universities, students choose different projects that require 'only' a survey because they mistakenly think that survey research is easy. Many graduates see evaluation as a major hurdle in the system development life cycle. Many are overwhelmed by the variety of studies that can be conducted and their associated statistical analysis. Reviewers perform poor (or erroneous!) reviews of programs and studies because they do not understand the design of studies. Recently, one of our students had a paper returned where one of the reviewers did not know the meaning of a 'quasi-experiment' and stated this in the review. It was clear that many questions this reviewer posed would have been answered if he had known the meaning of that term. Even more frustrating is that studies meant to evaluate software sometimes fail to show effects because the study was not properly designed, which is a waste of money and talent. In other cases, designers rely on effects that are untrustworthy because the study was not designed properly. Finally, many instructors in informatics do not include user studies in their courses because there is a lack of sufficient, high quality and comprehensive teaching materials to use as a base. And although few courses include this topic, quality journals and funding sources require it and all software would benefit from it.

In short, this book explains what an experimenter who is serious about evaluating an information system, be it a student, developer or researcher, should pay attention to and why. A good, trustworthy evaluation of an information system is a valuable activity that contributes to the bottom line. It does not have to be extremely expensive or time consuming but should be to the point and support moving the system development forward by providing informed choices. Proper evaluation leads to better information systems and can demonstrate their strengths and weaknesses.

Well designed user studies are a vital ingredient for success in informatics.

January 16, 2011   Gondy Leroy

Acknowledgements

Over the years I have worked with many doctoral students and reviewed numerous drafts for publications or grant proposals which showed me the breadth and depth of our field and allowed me to see the passion of developers and researchers to make a positive impact. It's been an honor and privilege to comment on and help improve those products and research projects. Being a first-hand witness to avoidable struggles and problems persuaded me to write this book. I had fun writing it and hope it will be useful to everyone who evaluates algorithms and information systems.

A brief word is needed to thank the many people who helped and supported me in writing this book.

First and foremost, I owe special thanks to Lorne Olfman (Claremont Graduate University) for his insightful comments, inquisitive questions and helpful suggestions after reviewing each chapter. It takes a lot of dedication and was also invaluable in helping me stick to my deadlines. Many thanks also to Byron Marshall (Oregon State University) for his thoughtful critiques and comments and for invariably pointing out another perspective so as to help me broaden the content. I owe thanks to Cynthia LeRouge (St. Louis University) for sharing experiences and IRB protocols and for her unbridled enthusiasm that was always encouraging. Thanks also to Charles V. Brown, Jr. (Charles Brown Healthcare) whose conversations over the years inspired several examples throughout the book. Last but not least, I want to thank Sarah Marshall for the excellent, timely and meticulous editing.

January 16, 2011   Gondy Leroy

Contents

Part I

Designing the User Study

Overview

1

Chapter Summary

This chapter provides an overview of different types of evaluation studies and their advantages and disadvantages. The studies that are reviewed range from naturalistic observations to controlled experiments. They differ in the amount of intervention by researchers and the degree to which the environment is controlled. For each, examples from the literature are included as illustrations.

Since this book focuses on the controlled experiment, the main section of the chapter provides an overview of the essential elements in such controlled experiments: the research hypotheses, the different types of variables that need to be defined, the sampling units which can be people or artifacts in informatics, random assignment and, finally, statistical analyses that allow generalization of a conclusion from a sample to a population. Although the examples in this and subsequent chapters are taken from the medical field, the study design methods are generic. As such, the content is applicable to the evaluation of information systems in other domains.

This chapter concludes with specific advice for conducting evaluation studies in a healthcare setting. Because this is a safety first field, special cautions and obstacles exist to ensure that no undue influence is exercised over the medical decision process and that no hazards or unhealthy situations are imposed on study participants.

Study Focus

Defining the study goal is important when designing any study. The goal guides both the development of an algorithm or information system and the evaluation. By focusing on the system, stakeholders and the timeline, the goal of the study can be clearly and completely defined. This allows the researcher to choose the best comparison conditions for the new system and so the definition of the independent variables: the conditions or treatments that are evaluated. In addition, with a clearly

G. Leroy, *Designing User Studies in Informatics*, Health Informatics,
DOI 10.1007/978-0-85729-622-1_1, © Springer-Verlag London Limited 2011

defined goal, the system's use goals can be better defined and its impact can be evaluated. This will lead to the definition of the dependent variables: the outcomes of using or implementing the new system.

System Focus

An information system is developed for a purpose: improvement in a process, an outcome, a situation or a person. The potential impact of the system should be defined and delineated so that the study can focus on evaluating whether the system fulfills this purpose.

For example, assume that a software developer proposes to develop an online system where patients can sign up for their appointment, read about what they can expect and how to prepare, and make changes to their appointment time. The system sends a reminder of the appointment a day in advance. The overall goal of this system is to reduce the number of no-shows in the clinic. The rationale is that by showing the schedule online and involving the patient as a partner in a conversation, the number of no-shows will lower. The clinic currently has no online presence but reminds people of their appointment by phone. The goal of the new system is very clear, so the evaluation should focus on measuring progress toward this goal. This has consequences for the study design. First of all, the conditions to be tested are the old and new system. These will be the two levels of the independent variable. One outcome to be tested is the number of no-shows. An additional outcome of interest is the number of changed appointment times. These will define the dependent variables. Additional measures can be included that may help understand the results or improve the system, but any evaluation that does not include the count of no-shows would be irrelevant.

Stakeholder Focus

Information systems affect people. Therefore, keeping the goals of these stakeholders in mind will further improve the study. The answers to essential questions such as "For whom is the study conducted?", "For what will the evaluation be used?" and even "What are the consequences and for whom?" will help with the design of the study. The stakeholders can change over time and over the course of the system's development. The example of the online appointments is used to illustrate the questions.

If the study is conducted early on in the development process, the goal may be to find out major obstacles. In this case, involving the developers will be very beneficial. The study may focus on an individual component instead of an entire system. In the example, an essential component for reducing the no-shows at the clinic would be a zero-learning time user interface. This may be the most important component of the entire system. Studies that are conducted later in the development cycles will focus on other outcomes that are more comprehensive. For example, the new appointment system may be installed and used for a trial period. The goal of an evaluation at this point would be to study the effects over a longer period of time of the reduction in no-shows and also the changes in appointments or popular appointment times. Keeping the future in mind, cost will be an important consideration and should be compared against the system that already was in place, in this case the phone calls. Such an evaluation also needs to be longitudinal, since the upfront costs may be high but the returned decrease in costs due to fewer no-shows may be steady or even increasing.

If stakeholders are mostly interested in this particular system, the study should focus on only the one implementation and clinic. However, if the stakeholders also are interested in expanding the system to different environments, additional measures can be included that shed light on how well it could be transported to such different places. Users' behaviors, attitudes, likes and dislikes, and intentions also will become important and may have to be included in the variables to be measured.

Timeline and Software Development Cycle

Modern software development approaches are ideally suited to integrate early testing of individual components. The entire product benefits from identifying and fixing problems in the early phases. This is not a luxury but a necessity, because today's information systems are complex, containing many integrated components. The components are usually developed separately, over different stages, by different people and need to be integrated to form the final system. When evaluations are delayed and conducted toward the end of the software development, it becomes increasingly difficult to pinpoint which components cause difficulty or which contribute most to success. The development cycle emphasizes gradual and modular development with the opportunity to backtrack and make corrections. This makes it possible to start testing and catch problems early, even at the design phase. In particular, problems that require changes in the underlying architecture of a system can be corrected much more easily in the beginning than later on, when the component has been integrated in the complete system. Such architectural changes late in the development cycle will require nearly all components to be adjusted.

The benefits of early testing are more easily demonstrated by pointing to problems resulting from lack of testing. Most defects originate in the requirements analysis phase, but the majority (60%) of them are not detected until user acceptance testing [1], demonstrating the importance of testing early and frequently. The problems often result from a lack of communication [2] leading to misunderstood requirements [3] and products that do not match user expectations. User studies like those described in this book are suited to uncovering such problems with expectations and misunderstood requirements. Research on gathering user requirements has clearly shown the increased costs associated with fixing problems later in the development stages. The lack of testing contributes to very costly software, since correcting mistakes becomes nearly exponentially more expensive in later development phases: up to 100–200 times higher after implementation than when detected during requirements gathering [2, 4, 5].

Developers have many reasons for avoiding early testing. None are valid. Early testing is sometimes seen as a waste of time, but there are good software tools available that make early testing of user interfaces and even underlying algorithms possible. Software development kits (SDK), such as the Java Development Kit (JDK), make it easy to add a graphical user interface (GUI). Such a GUI can be added to an algorithm to facilitate showing its output in real time in a user friendly manner, even if the GUI will never be reused again. Furthermore, object oriented or modular design facilitates testing and improving individual components. Then, early testing is sometimes seen as taking too much time away from the design and development team. However, early testing helps evaluate components and can help define, improve and fine-tune them. This helps clarify the goals of using the system. Given the difficulty encountered with extracting user requirements, any clarification will be beneficial. A well designed study will also try to answer specific questions that developers may have which would otherwise be answers with best guesses, not facts. A final reason that leads to avoiding testing is the lack of expertise and experience with software evaluation. This book provides the background information needed to conduct such studies.

In medical informatics, the decisions resulting from studies are often labeled differently depending on the type of evaluation that was done: formative versus summative [6, 7]. *Formative evaluations*, also called *constructive evaluations*, are evaluations of an information system that are conducted during the design process. These evaluations are executed before the product has been finalized and often aim to provide direction for future development. For example, usability studies are often conducted as formative studies to inform the design process on interface design and user expectations. When problems are discovered early, they can be corrected and the product can be improved. Such formative studies fit very well in iterative software development processes. In contrast, *summative evaluations* are studies conducted after all development has been completed and the information system has been placed in its intended environment. These studies are meant to be a final evaluation of the system and its objectives. Summative evaluations may be longitudinal, as the use of systems may change once they have been in place for a period of time. However, if the system performs as intended, results from the different studies should corroborate each other.

Depending on the stage of development, different types of studies can be conducted. Even before a particular system is designed, observational studies may be done to learn about an environment and the potential for improvement. Then, separate algorithms and systems need to be tested for speed, efficiency and correctness. For example, when developing a medical records system, each component and each connection between components must be tested. Every study design has strengths and weaknesses. Some are faster and easier to do, but they are less representative of the actual context where the system will be placed. Others are very difficult to do but may lead to extremely valuable data. Naturally, the difficulty of a study does not make it better. Understanding user study design also means that one can conduct the studies to maximize the impact. There is not one magic formula that can be used to decide which study should be conducted for different systems in different development phases. Ideally, multiple studies are conducted during the development phase and after completion of the system. Each will provide a different view on the use of the software. However, only one type of study allows for causal conclusions. That is the controlled experiment, also called the controlled randomized trial. It is the topic of this book and it will be referred to, in short, as 'the user study'. The person conducting the study is referred to as the 'researcher'.

Study Types

Many different evaluation study types exist. Not all are suitable to evaluate software and no single approach is perfect. In reality, using a multi-study approach during the design, development and installation of information systems is best. It will provide better insight and high quality data. However, in many fields, and especially in medical informatics, there is a focus on randomized trials, the type of user studies described in this book. As Kaplan [8] points out, since physicians are often encouraged to evaluate information systems in the same manner as new drugs and reviewers of publications place higher value on controlled studies, fewer studies of different types can be found in this field.

The different types of studies vary in their intensity of observation and interaction with the observed environment. In addition, the researcher's focus can be on one aspect or multiple aspects of the environment, on one actor or multiple actors and can be more or less interventional.

Naturalistic Observation

When a study takes the form of a *naturalistic observation*, the researcher studies the individuals in their natural setting. The researcher does not intrude and no changes are introduced in the environment to compare differences in behaviors or opinions. It is a passive form of research. Ideally, people are not aware of the observation so that they do not change their behaviors. The study method provides rich datasets but is usually limited in the number of observations that can be made. Each observation requires a significant investment of the observer's time and effort. Observers are present and continuously code behaviors of interest. For example, Tesh and Holditch-Davis [9] worked with three observers who watched the interactions between mothers and their prematurely born babies to evaluate two instruments, the Nursing Child Assessment Teaching Scale (NCATS) and the Home Observation for Measurement of the Environment (HOME) inventory, and relate them to the interactive behaviors that they observed.

Today's abundance of video cameras for recording behaviors and the increasing comfort of people with being videotaped have led to a somewhat different flavor of naturalistic observation. It has made observing without intervening significantly easier. For example, Lambrechts et al. [10] used video recording to study the reaction of clinical staff to aggressive and self-injurious behaviors of individuals with severe intellectual disabilities. Although a video recording may be seen as intrusive and causing changes in behavior, for many people, their awareness of the recording disappears quickly and normal behavior resumes. Campos et al. [11] used naturalistic observation to study the family interaction of dual-earner families. They videotaped adults and children in their home environment for 2 weekdays. Analysis was done based on these video recordings.

Case Studies, Field Studies and Descriptive Studies

Several types of studies fall under this heading and several flavors of each type also exist where some intervention by researchers is incorporated in the study. What all these studies have in common is that they help explain and answer difficult questions. They can help find an answer to key questions such as "Why was the system not accepted?" and "How could it have led to incorrect decisions?" [12]. They also are suited to consider several characteristics of work environment, culture, lifestyle and personal preferences when searching for explanations. In contrast, these characteristics are systematically controlled in experiments and so cannot easily contribute to a more complete explanation. These studies can also be combined with action research.

Case studies analyze one system or one person. The researcher observes select behaviors over time. The goal of doing a *descriptive study* is to evaluate one or more variables with a set of participants. Friedman describes subjective studies as following an "illuminative/responsive approach to evaluation" (page 205) [6]. A *field study* is somewhat broader in that normal activities are studied in their normal environment [13]. Field studies are ideal for longitudinal research, since normal activities can be followed and evaluated. Similar to a case study, a field study can generate very rich data. Special analysis, such as systematic content analysis of study notes, is needed to manage and interpret the data.

The studies in this category are ideal when complemented with surveys and controlled experiments. Surveys result in correlations between variables and experiments in causal relationships. In both, effects are commonly observed but not explained. Case studies, field studies and descriptive studies can help explain. This is especially the case with survey research where there are often many significant correlations that tell only part of the story. Similarly, it is not unusual for a post hoc analysis of experiment data to show unexpected effects. It is often difficult to understand why these effects exist, or who or what is responsible. Case studies and descriptive studies can provide answers to such questions. They are excellent vehicles to follow experiments and help understand the phenomena that were observed. But they also can play a complementary role and lead to interesting research hypotheses that can be studied by conducting experiments.

One variable commonly tested in information systems research as part of these types of studies is user acceptance. For example, Purkis [14] describes a case study conducted in Canada with nursing staff. A center was being established where nurses would work with the community in a different manner than the customary interactions in hospitals. The goal was to allow nurses to work to their full extent, without being held back by common hospital guidelines and while not duplicating services. These activities needed to be documented using new information technology. The researchers worked with the nurses on an information system for recording activities, worked through problems recording that information and identified the consequences of using the information technology.

Action Research

Action-case research [7] or *action research* [15] combines approaches from case studies but includes direct involvement of the researcher. With this approach, the researcher is less of an observer but instead takes an incremental, iterative and error-correcting approach [7]. A common element between action research and case or field studies is the immersion of the researcher in the environment where the study takes place. Similar to the previously discussed studies, this immersion offers the opportunity to study difficult questions related to the *why* and *how* of events. However, there are also significant differences from those study types.

A first difference between action research and other immersive approaches is the goal of the research. The goal is to solve a problem or improve an existing situation. For example, Boursnell and Prosser [16] applied the action research methodology to increase awareness about domestic violence in women and children. In their study for Emergency Room (ER) personnel, a Violence, Abuse and Neglect Prevention Team collaborated with nurses in the ER departments. Discussions and trainings were held in such a manner that all participants took ownership of the project and results. The study led to a survey tool to help identify domestic violence victims that included both pre- and post-implementation survey based evaluations which showed an increase in awareness of the problem and increased confidence in addressing it. An additional file audit showed a change in behaviors during and after the project.

A second difference is the type of interaction with study participants. In most studies, the participants are called the *subjects* of the study. They are the people who are subjected to study methods. In contrast, people who partake in action research are intended to become active participants in the project [15]. The researchers act more as facilitators than as experts or observers. The participants are more involved in the project; their role is not reduced to receiving a treatment. For example, in Norway, Borg et al. [17] adopted an action research approach to learn about and help improve a homecare model being pioneered. The goal of the homecare model was to minimize hospitalizations. To this end, mental health clinicians formed crisis resolution and home treatment teams. At the onset of this initiative, the researchers conducted multi-stage focus groups where they facilitated the meetings to discuss the team workings, collect data and support the clinical teams in developing best practices for their interventions.

A third difference is that action researchers focus on a particular problem or project and will actively try to influence what is happening. Because of this active nature, action research also is more cyclical than the other study types. Researchers will plan an action by looking at relevant information and building a picture; then they will think about possible actions and conduct the actions together with the participants. This cycle can be repeated multiple times. For example, Butera-Prinzi et al. [18] describe an Australian action research project aiming to improve the long term care provided for persons with acquired brain injury, and their family life and family outlook. Using an action research approach, seven facilitators and 96 participating family members collaborated in a structured approach toward the development of a process of face-to-face and teleconference family linkups that were intended to provide social support. In a cyclical process, several linkup sessions were conducted and evaluated by both the facilitators and participants. The facilitators also met separately over a 12 month period to discuss and improve the process.

Finally, in addition to taking action, the researcher also evaluates the effects of the actions. Although this research focuses on action, there also is room to interpret results and difficulties and explain these as part of theorizing, which helps broaden the context of the lessons learned. As the many examples in the literature demonstrate, the level and amount of activity in action research varies and is adjusted to the individual projects. What is noteworthy in all these projects is that, when they are conducted well, very practical lessons are learned. These lessons may not be applicable to every possible situation, but the available information on the context and reasons for moving forward make it possible for others to extract relevant advice and benefit even if the projects are not closely related.

Action research is not as common as other study types in medicine, but it may be of particular value to the medical field because of its central tenet, which is to bring changes that have a positive social value [19] and that keep people's well-being in mind [15]. It is furthermore a flexible approach to research. The researcher keeps the context in mind and adjusts the planned interventions accordingly. One such example of trying to foster positive social values is the work by Delobelle et al. [20] in Africa. They are applying action research to transform a study hospital in rural South Africa into a Health Promoting Hospital (HPH). HPHs are seen as active systems that involve the community, their staff and patients in improving healthcare, living and working conditions and increasing satisfaction of all stakeholders.

Surveys

A *survey* is a list of questions or statements about study elements of interest distributed to large groups of people. Surveys are useful to measure opinions, intentions, feelings and beliefs, among others. They also can be very useful instruments to establish whether a product can fulfill a need, help solve a problem or determine its probable future popularity. Well constructed surveys, however, are designed to minimize bias and to ensure that they measure what they claim they measure; the measurements are reliable and results can be generalized both toward a larger population and also over time. Several books exist to help design and validate surveys based on item response theory, classical test theory and others [21–24]. For example, test–retest evaluation, item analysis and factor analysis on results for an entire survey are needed to design a valid and reliable survey. Such validated surveys are a good basis for correlation studies. When they are part of a comprehensive user study that includes additional measures, these surveys also often capture very valuable qualitative data essential to understanding the study results. However, it is essential to take into account that even the best surveys have many potential problems [7].

Although constructing a survey and distributing it may seem easy and fast, in reality, this is a misconception. Many researchers rely on hastily put together surveys that have not been validated. While these may be nice add-ons to other measures in controlled experiments and a quick way to get feedback, such surveys should not be the main basis for drawing conclusions. Many studies include an ad hoc survey to evaluate satisfaction of participants. These surveys have limited value. There is an enormous difference between these custom-designed surveys and standardized and validated surveys. Since no measurement studies (see below) have been conducted on such ad hoc surveys, it is uncertain what exactly is being measured. In addition, there is no information about suspected biases that may influence the results, or to what extent the information may be incomplete or inconclusive.

Some common problems with hastily put together surveys affect their usefulness. Respondents may misunderstand the intent or the meaning of the survey items. When they do not understand the statement as intended, no trustworthy conclusions can be drawn from the responses. These problems result from the language used in the survey items. Especially for participants with limited literacy skills, items may be too difficult to understand. Phrasing items is even more complicated because they also have to be neutral and focused on one aspect at a time. When a question is not neutral, it may indicate approval or disapproval of an opinion and participants may be influenced by this in their answer. When multiple aspects are included, it is unclear to which one a participant is responding. For example, a statement such as "Do you intend to walk at least 1 h and eat one serving of fruit per day?" should be split into two separate statements.

In addition, respondents will always answer from their own context and so emotions, past experiences and prejudices will all influence the answers. Relying on survey results for measurement of behaviors or actions is dangerous because all surveys rely on self-reporting. This leads to a set of potential problems such as bias, guessing and even dishonesty. Many people have good intentions and fully intend to do the right thing when given the opportunity. But actual behaviors are often different from intentions. Surveys are good for measuring intentions, but do not allow conclusions about actual behaviors. Not all participants will be honest when filling out a survey, especially with regard to sensitive questions related to sexual conduct, income or lifestyle. Furthermore, survey respondents often have to rely on their memory of events and this may introduce another set of biases or outright errors. For example, answers to common questions in the doctor's office about the amount of alcoholic drinks consumed on average tend to be underestimates.

Although the points mentioned above may seem obvious, many surveys include mistakes along these lines. Constructing a good survey is difficult and time consuming. For example, Rushton et al. [25] went through several cycles to develop and validate a seemingly simple survey to measure confidence in using wheel chairs. Fischer et al. [26] demonstrate the problems with survey research. They used a construct in the Canadian Alcohol and Drug Use Monitoring Survey to measure non-prescription opioid usage in Canada. The results showed rates so much lower than expected that the researchers question the survey approach to get this type of data. They point out that responders' memory problems, dishonesty and a different interpretation of specific survey items may have led to the results. Unfortunately, in both informatics and medicine, surveys are often constructed in an ad hoc manner. Jaussent et al. [27] reviewed 21 surveys in French and English that are intended to measure healthcare professionals' knowledge, perceptions and practices related to alcoholism. They concluded that the surveys were often lacking in quality and that the most important properties, validity, reliability and sensitivity, are often ignored. They also point out that many surveys lack a theoretical background.

Correlation Studies

Correlation studies are used to describe changes in variables. In particular, their goal is to find where change in one variable coincides with change in another. Correlation studies usually involve looking at many variables and many data points for each variable. They often rely on surveys and large population samples. However, it is important to understand that these studies do not attempt to discover what causes a change. When two variables A and B are found to correlate with each other, this does not show whether A caused B, B caused A, or whether there was a third factor causing both A and B to change. Correlation studies do not investigate the direction of the relation. Attribution of causation to a correlation is a common mistake made by laymen and beginning researchers. For example, when reading online health community blogs, several examples can be found where this relation is misunderstood. Bloggers relate co-occurring events and mistake them as causing each other. Sometimes, this error is pointed out by others bloggers, but often it leads to more bloggers bringing additional anecdotal evidence testifying to the assumed causal effect.

Although controlled experiments and surveys are considered very different, they have several elements in common. Both often have the same goal, namely the testing of a research hypothesis. The goal then is to find relations between suspected influential variables and a certain outcome. The outcome is the actual variable of interest. The other variables are expected to influence this outcome. These influences can be a variety of things, such as treatments received, environmental conditions and personal characteristics of people. The main difference between a correlation study and an experiment is that in a correlation study, the different levels of the influential variables cannot be randomly assigned to groups of people and people cannot be randomly assigned to conditions. For example, gender may be a very important factor, but people cannot be randomly assigned to the male or female group. Correlation research has to work with the data as it is received. Correlation studies measure many variables of which the different levels have not been randomly assigned to participants. After measurements, the correlations are calculated between the outcome and the other potentially influential characteristics. The researcher looks at the relations between the measured levels of the variables and the outcome, which can be very educational and helpful in forming or disproving a theory. However, since it is not possible to randomly assign people to a condition or treatment level of a variable, a correlation study cannot draw causal conclusions. Because two items correlate, one does not necessarily cause the other. In many cases, there will be a third factor causing both.

In medicine, correlation studies often form the start for new research. Correlations are frequently discovered between measurements and outcomes. The relations are interesting but the underlying cause has not been explained, hence the need for more research. For example, Palmirotta et al. [28] describe the association between Birt Hogg Dube syndrome and cancer predisposition. It is not given that one causes the other. Instead, both may be due to the same underlying genetic mutations. In informatics, correlation studies are often used to evaluate technology acceptance in circumstances where controlled experiments are impractical. In these cases, one of two theories often form the starting point: Theory of Planned Behavior (TPB) by Ajzen [29] or the Technology Acceptance Model (TAM) by Davis [30]. According to the TPB, intentions to behave in a certain way can be predicted with accuracy from attitudes towards the behavior, subjective norms and perceived behavioral control. For example, Hu et al. [31, 32] based their research on the TPB to evaluate the acceptance of telemedicine by physicians. They concluded that the physicians' attitudes towards the new technology and the perceived risk of using the technology are important factors in the adoption process. However, many more variables can be studied. According to the TAM, system usage can be predicted based on the usefulness and ease of use with attitude and intention as mediating variables. In a comparative study, both models were able to predict the same behavior [33] with comparable accuracy.

Measurement Studies

Measurement studies are a special kind of study that are different from experiments or demonstration studies [6], which are the topic of this book. The goal of a measurement study is to define and validate measures of an attribute. In other words, it is a study that helps develop and validate the metrics that will be used in demonstration studies. A measurement of a person's or system's characteristics with a metric provides an observed value. This observed value consists of the actual value and some error. Measurement studies aim to design measurements that have little error variance and a known error rate. Note that this goal is similar to demonstration studies, where proper design can help reduce variance in measurement due to error. With numerous scales and tools being automated and put online for use via websites or mobile devices, these measurement studies are very important. For example, Honeth et al. [34] compared an Internet based hearing test with an accepted gold standard. Before such a new test can be accepted, the authors needed to show that the results are as valid and reliable as the accepted gold standard. Ives et al. [35] conducted a large scale evaluation of an existing and validated survey to measure 'user information satisfaction'. Unfortunately, such thorough evaluations are the exception more than the rule in informatics.

When the measurement studies have shown a metric to be valuable and valid, these metrics can be used in demonstration studies. Ideally, any metric used in a demonstration study should have been shown to be reliable and valid in a measurement study. *Reliability* refers to the ability to repeat the measurement and achieve the same results because the degree of random noise in a measurement remains low [6]. When there is a lot of random noise, measurements will vary for no good reason and are not reliable. *Validity* refers to the idea that the items being used measure what was intended to be measured. With an invalid measurement, there is misdirection: something else is being measured. In psychology, for example, where new scales are often developed to measure psychological constructs, validity is partially evaluated by relating the new measure to an existing one for which the validity has already been shown. With the increasing use of computer applications that allow self-administration, either online or via another means, there is much need to assess the new informatics-enabled surveys to ensure that results achieved with the computer version of a test are similar to the paper–pencil version or can be translated such that the same standards can be used. A good example of such comparison is the work by Chinman et al. [36], who evaluated a computer-assisted self-interviewing approach to conducting assessments for patients with schizophrenia or bipolar disorder. They compared assessments gained with a standard Revised Behavior and Symptom Identification Scale (R-BASIC) and with an online self-paced version. Subjects completed both assessments and the results were compared for internal consistency, validity, bias and usability. The consistency and validity were comparable, no bias was introduced and the online version was preferred by the participants.

Quasi-Experiments

Quasi-experiments differ from experiments in their lack of randomization. Subjects are not randomly assigned to conditions. In many cases, randomization is impossible because of practical or ethical reasons. Adopting a quasi-experiment design does not necessarily mean that the study will be simpler, and although the shortcomings are substantial, quasi-experiments often yield valuable, high quality information. When conducting quasi-experiments, much attention should be paid to the potential systematic bias that may be introduced and which will, if present, influence the results. For example, when one group of patients gets a new treatment and the other groups get the *old* treatment, this may lead to differences in motivation and attention being paid, different behaviors by both groups and even resentment for receiving the old treatment.

Quasi-experiments are often conducted for a comparison between different groups that cannot be split up, for groups that exist at different time periods, when randomization is not seen as ethical or fair, or for other practical limitations such as geographical constraints, social constraints (e.g., use of family units) and time constraints. The three constraints are discussed below. Example studies were included to illustrate the constraints, even though some did not include information technology. Naturally, other reasons than these three exist.

Geographical constraints on the randomization process are practical obstacles that cannot be overcome because distances are too large or because it is impossible to control different conditions within one geographical unit. A good example is the study by Sunaert et al. [37, 38] that describes a quasi-experiment in Belgium to evaluate improving chronic care for patients with Type 2 diabetes. Two geographical regions, comparable in terms of socio-economic characteristics and healthcare facilities, were chosen. The same inclusion/exclusion criteria were used in both regions to select patients. In the intervention region, changes in the healthcare system were implemented during a 4 year action research project. Information technology, a registration database, was used in a limited way. The intervention focused on improving coordination and continuity of care and increasing patient support. Within-subject comparisons were made based on time: the same subjects were measured before and after the intervention. Between-subject comparisons were made between existing regions: subjects in the intervention and control region were compared. Assignment to the intervention or control depended on geography, not random assignment. Overall, the two groups were comparable in terms of their socio-demographic characteristics – just one characteristic was significantly different between the two groups – making it easier to exclude possible confounding variables. Several significant effects were found between the groups and within each group over time, leading to a rich evaluation. Although the study did not focus solely on information technology, it is an excellent example of how a quasi-experiment can unearth obstacles to using technology and pinpoint the specific tools that could augment and make better use of the available electronic medical records.

Social constraints can exist in many different forms. A common form is when children are the participants in a study. It may be difficult to randomly assign children from the same family to different experimental conditions. Doing this may introduce different types of bias and could be worse than using a quasi-experimental design. Other types of social organizations, religious groups, schools or sports teams in our society may lead to the same constraints on experimental design. For example, Herz et al. [39] studied the impact of sex education on inner-city, seventh- and eighth-grade students. The researchers worked with an experimental and control school from which students were randomly selected. Pre- and post-tests were used to evaluate the impact of the intervention, which consisted of 15 sessions on topics such as reproductive anatomy, conception, contraception and pregnancy, as well as developing career goals.

Sometimes, controlled experiments cannot be conducted because of *time constraints*, for example, when the control group consists of an older generation. In these cases, a quasi-experimental design allows for more comparisons than a single condition study could provide. This is especially the case when studies take a long time, historical data is already available and researchers have access to that archived data. Instead of conducting a completely new experiment, the conditions of the archived data can be taken into account, making it possible to link the new study with the archived study through the design of a quasi-experiment. Especially when introducing new information systems, where previously there were none, these quasi-experiments can provide much needed and high quality data. These also are called *historically-controlled experiments* [6]. For example, when Glynn et al. [40] were comparing an online psycho-educational program for relatives of people with schizophrenia, they compared the results of their online intervention with data from previous family therapy interventions. Kröncke [41] compared computer based education versus participation in a laboratory experiment: one cohort of second-year medical students received the computer tool; the other cohort of second-year medical students participated in the laboratory experiment.

Quasi experiments may give an indication of the results to expect, but caution is needed for generalization because of the biases that cannot be controlled. For example, participants' knowledge that one is receiving a new treatment versus an old treatment will affect the outcome. Other factors that may not have been randomized may affect the outcome too. For example, there may be practical reasons why participants are in specific groups. Children may be put in the same classroom because they all need to take the bus home instead of walking home, which would probably be a reflection of demographic differences. High performers may have been put in one classroom, which would reflect differences in a possible host of factors. Undecided students may have taken longer to sign up for classes and they may be together in groups for that reason. Such non-random groups will often display systematically different characteristics between groups. The researcher is often unaware of them or does not have the means to correct for them.

In conclusion, it is clear that the convenience of existing groups makes quasi-experimental studies very useful. Many of the potential differences can be measured allowing the differences between the groups to be documented. As long as researchers understand the shortcomings of a quasi-experimental design, they can be careful not to over-generalize the findings, measure differences to demonstrate where control and experimental groups differ, and so bring a rich dataset and valuable conclusions to the community.

Controlled Experiments or Demonstration Studies

The user studies discussed in this book are also called *demonstration studies, controlled experiments, randomized controlled trials*, or *comparative studies* in medical informatics [6]. The goal of the studies is to evaluate hypotheses about causal relations between variables. In the case of informatics, these studies evaluate the impact, benefit, advantages, disadvantages or other effects of information systems. The new or improved system is compared to other systems or under different conditions and evaluated for its impact.

To speak of an experiment, several elements need to be in place. Each is discussed in detail in the following chapters. First, the researcher must manipulate one or more variables. These are the independent variables. Second, these variables must be chosen in response to the research questions and hypotheses. In other words, a good study will have clear goals for the evaluation to be undertaken and should focus on providing the missing knowledge. Third, the researcher must control sources of error and undesired variance as much as possible. These requirements are discussed in the next part under nuisance variables. Fourth, and most importantly, the sampling units of the study, usually participants or data representing people, have to be randomly assigned to the experimental conditions. Fifth, the experimenter must specify who the subjects will be, which population they represent and how many subjects should make up the study sample so that the sample is a reasonable representation of the population. And finally, the necessary statistical analyses should be conducted to test whether there were any effects.

There are many examples of experiments in the literature and, since they are the topic of this book, many are highlighted throughout the text.

Study Elements

When designing a user study, there are five important elements, as defined by Kirk [42], that need to be taken into consideration and that are essential in an experiment in the behavioral sciences and also in user studies in informatics. Although user studies in informatics are usually simpler than those in behavioral sciences, e.g., the outcomes that are measured are often more straightforward, these elements are still required and should be taken into account when designing the study. Only after careful consideration of each element can one design a valid and useful user study.

Hypotheses

The first essential element is the formulation of hypotheses. Formulating hypotheses helps one focus the study and choose the best metrics. To formulate the hypotheses, it is necessary to clearly define the goal of the information system or intervention. For example, a researcher's goal may be to increase patient understanding of a medical procedure such as coronary angioplasty. This goal was established after it became clear that educational pamphlets available in the hospital were insufficient. The researcher believes that a 3D video showing the procedure would be a much better solution because it can let a person *see* how the procedure is done. In this example, the research hypothesis is that a 3D movie fragment will increase health literacy more than the available text.

Once the research hypothesis is clear, it needs to be translated into a hypothesis that can be statistically tested. Statistical hypotheses are formulated to specify a test of the scientific hypotheses; they are the testable version. When evaluating information systems, the research and statistical hypotheses are usually closely related. For example, one could hypothesize that the patient's score on a quiz about coronary angioplasty is higher for those patients who watched the 3D video compared to the patients who read the pamphlet. Clearly, there are many factors that can contribute to a difference in patient understanding in this study. The text may include information not covered in the video or more time may be spent reading and studying the text than watching the video. To avoid unclear or biased results and make it possible to draw a conclusion, several variables, such as the amount of information and the allowed study time, need to be defined and controlled.

Variables

The second essential element to consider in a user study consists of the variables. Several types of variables, discussed later in this part, need to be considered: the independent variable, the dependent variable and the nuisance variables. The independent variable is what is manipulated and controlled by the investigator. In the behavioral sciences, the independent variable could consist of levels of the treatment of interest. For example, in psychology, it could be negative versus positive reinforcement of a behavior; in medicine, it could be levels of radiation or different drug regimes. In informatics, the independent variable focuses on the information system or algorithm that is being evaluated. The independent variable could be the presence or absence of a system, different versions of a system or a comparison of an old versus a new system.

The dependent variable is the measurement that is recorded and used to evaluate the independent variable. When only one dependent variable is considered at a time, the analysis is called *univariate* analysis. In contrast, when multiple dependent variables are considered together, this is called *multivariate* analysis. In multivariate analysis, multiple variables are considered together and a mathematical model is tested that describes the means and the covariation between the variables [43], sometimes over longer time periods [44]. This book focuses on univariate analysis and assumes that only one dependent variable is considered at a time. When multiple dependent variables are of interest, they are evaluated independently from each other. In informatics, the dependent variable is most often straightforward. For example, a multiple choice test on coronary angioplasty could be used to evaluate the patients' knowledge of the procedure. This could be done after each intervention, the text and the video. In the example above, the outcomes of the test need to be compared to evaluate the effect of the 3D video.

A third variable that cannot be ignored is the nuisance variable. Nuisance variables influence the outcome of a study but are not the main interest of the study. For example, some patients may have significantly more knowledge about coronary angioplasty, making it difficult to rely on a one time measurement using the multiple choice task. Other patients may have limited depth perception, e.g., due to amblyopia, and so cannot benefit as much from a 3D video. Nuisance variables that systematically influence a dependent variable introduce bias. Being aware of these variables makes it possible to control them. For example, a pre-test could disqualify patients who have knowledge of coronary angioplasty. Alternatively, patients could take a multiple choice pre-test to measure their starting knowledge of coronary angioplasty. The experimenter could look for additional information learned from reading the text or watching the video, and the dependent variable could be the increase of knowledge as measured by the increase in items correctly answered between the pre- and post-test, in other words, by subtracting the pre-treatment score from the post-treatment score. Naturally, this introduces a new bias, namely that people may be more likely to give the same answer to a question the second time they are asked it. This illustrates the need for careful consideration of all possible nuisance variables when conducting a study.

Study Participants and Other Sampling Units

The third necessary element when designing a user study is the specification of the sampling units. In experimental studies, the number of observations depends on the sampling units. In the informatics studies discussed here, such sampling units can be a variety of things. They can be human participants whose task performance, opinions, behaviors, or attitudes are measured. They also can be artifacts created or generated by humans, such as text messages, outcomes on diagnostic tests or diagnostic images. In most of the studies referenced in this book, the sampling units will be people, such as nurses, physicians, patients, consumers; or groups of people, such as departments and support groups. However, since an evaluation of algorithms also can be conducted as a user study, the sampling units may be artifacts created by people, for example, personal health records, and these can form the input for an algorithm or information system that is to be evaluated.

This element may be more complicated in medicine (see next section). However, it is important that the subjects are as representative as possible of the intended population. It is not very helpful to design a system for nurses and test it with graduate computer science students.

Random Assignment

This fourth element is the assignment of sampling units to the experimental conditions. To draw causal conclusions about an independent variable, it is essential that units are randomly assigned to experimental conditions. This random assignment is what differentiates a true experiment from a quasi-experiment. As will be shown with the experimental design model, there are always individual variations in each observation made. Each individual observation that belongs to a unit consists of multiple components, such as the true value and variation that is brought about by the experimental treatment, random noise and individual differences. When the participants are randomly distributed to treatments, these variations not due to the experimental manipulation can be expected to be randomly distributed and not systematically influence the results. This is also a main assumption of statistical analyses such as Analysis of Variance (ANOVA).

Random assignment does not give license to ignore nuisance variables. Assume for simplicity that the subjects in an experiment have either high or no knowledge of coronary angioplasty. In each group, half of the subjects would receive the text and the other half the 3D video based on a random decision process. Since these differences may vary significantly and affect the outcome of the study, the researcher could adjust the dependent variable to measure the increase in knowledge or could better define the study population as people with little or no knowledge about coronary angioplasty before starting the study. These are just two of the options at the researcher's disposal.

Statistical Analysis

Finally, the fifth essential characteristic of a well designed user study is a statistical analysis. This analysis is needed to determine whether a hypothesis, which relates the variables to each other, should be rejected or not. When an experiment is conducted, the researcher's goal is to decide whether a condition, such as a new information system, has an effect on a population of participants or artifacts. The user study is carried out with a sample of participants or artifacts intended to represent the entire population. The researcher's interest is not limited to that sample; he wants to find out if the conditions and its effect also would apply to the entire population. Statistical testing is necessary to make this jump. With appropriate testing, the researcher can make decisions about the population of interest based on the sample in the experiment.

Depending on the number of subjects that can be recruited and the number of treatments they participate in, the statistical tests will differ. T-tests are appropriate for studies where two conditions are compared. Analysis of variance (ANOVA) is most appropriate for studies where more than two conditions are compared. Variants for both these types of tests take into account how the sample of people or artifacts was assigned to the experimental conditions. For example, a paired samples t-test or a repeated measures ANOVA are appropriate when subjects participate in all experimental conditions. In other cases, the independent samples t-test or an ANOVA will be more appropriate. All these tests are discussed in later chapters.

Study Design Overview

In this section, a few main concepts about the design of a study are briefly introduced, including the difference between a sample and population, the normal distribution of scores of a population and how differences in distribution can indicate a significant effect of a treatment. Each is discussed in more detail in subsequent chapters.

Ultimately, the information systems that are being designed and developed are meant to be used by people. From a business perspective, it is usually the case that the more users there are the better. However, it is unpractical and often impossible to test an information system or its algorithms with all potential users. Therefore, it is necessary to rely on a sample of the entire population. Sample and population are two terms used in experimental design. *Population* stands for the entire group of users of interest. *Sample* stands for the smaller group of participants that is intended to represent the population. User studies and statistical tests are designed so that conclusions about the population can be drawn based on the results of experimenting on a sample. To ensure that the conclusions have the highest chance of being correct, the study must be well designed, participants must be representative and the sample must be large enough. The how-to is discussed in the subsequent chapters.

When conducting a study, the participants' scores on the variables of interest are collected. It is assumed that the frequency distribution of the scores will assume a bell shape (a normal distribution). This assumption can be tested and should be true for the statistical analysis to be valid. In general terms, this means that most people's scores will be close to each other with a few people having extreme answers. For example, when large enough samples of men are taken, their weight, height and intelligence will most likely be normally distributed. Similarly, when testing medical students on their knowledge of chemistry with a few questions, the average score will most probably be normally distributed. A normal distribution is a frequency distribution with special characteristics. The distribution is completely defined when the mean and the standard deviation are known and it allows conclusions about the probability of measuring a specific value. Normal distribution is an assumption of t-tests and ANOVA and is discussed in detail in subsequent chapters. Once the measurements are collected, they can be compared to establish whether the treatment, for example, the use of a new information system, made a difference or not. If that new system makes a difference, then the group of users with that system will score higher than the users without the system. Their scores will still be distributed normally, but, since they are shown to be different, they represent two different populations each with its own normal distribution. For example, if one developed an avatar based, personalized chemistry tutor for medical students, the group with the tutor would be expected to do better on their exams than the group without. Their mean score would be higher but there would still be about the same amount of variation in each group.

Designing a study well helps the researcher detect a difference, if it exists, between conditions. When the study is poorly designed and has many biases that are not controlled, the scores will show a lot of variation not due to the experimental treatment. The bell-shaped curves will be very broad and overlapping, and it will be unclear whether these two samples really belong to two different populations or just one. It will be hard to demonstrate that the differences in means exist. Statistical tests such as ANOVA incorporate these considerations by comparing the variance between groups with the variance within a group. Ideally, the variance between groups will be large, for example, a large benefit of using the chemistry tutor; and the variance within the group will be small, for example, everyone scores very high on the exams after using the tutor with little difference between people. A well designed study will also impact the number of participants that are needed to detect the effect. With an appropriate design and sample size, even very small effects can be detected with confidence. The following chapters include a discussion of the independent variables, their relations to the normal distribution and how statistical analysis can use that information to compare different treatments.

Special Considerations for Medical Informatics

The ultimate goal of using information technology in medicine is to improve health, healthcare and quality of life. The technology may be intended to do that directly, for example, by optimizing an intervention; but also indirectly, for example, by providing decision support and so improving diagnoses. Because studies in informatics focus on evaluating information systems and not, for example, attitudes, cognition or belief systems, the study designs are fairly straightforward: the goal is the improvement of a current situation and the evaluation is done to check whether this happened or not. Although care needs to be taken not to introduce bias and to ensure a fair evaluation, the outcomes can often be measured directly. This is different from other fields; for example, in psychology the constructs that are measured need to be derived from answers on surveys.

Although the study designs are straightforward, the execution of the studies can be more complicated because the field is medicine and healthcare. It is imperative that no harm is done. Because of this safety first principle, there are special considerations for conducting studies in medicine that complicate their execution. These range from ethical concerns to practical obstacles. Ammenwertha [45] suggests that the problems can be grouped in three categories: problems due to the complexity of what is being evaluated since information technology is not a simple object, problems due to the complexities associated with the process of evaluating in healthcare and problems associated with motivation to conduct a study. A few of these problems are highlighted below.

Study Subjects

Depending on the information technology being developed, the people participating in the user study can be individual clinicians, researchers, patients, consumers or groups of people. The information system is designed for a particular group and so should be evaluated by that group. It is essential that the study is conducted with a representative sample of users. This will ensure that the study conclusions apply to the population who are expected to buy, use and value the software. This is called external validity.

In medicine, involving the intended user is often difficult. If the intended users are medical doctors, it will be challenging to schedule studies because of their limited time availability. Finding a large group of them will be nearly impossible. One will need to convince the clinician that the system addresses an existing problem or can provide a marked improvement over existing systems. Once they have engaged clinicians, the researchers need to make sure to make the best use of the clinician's time. For example, it is not advised to have clinicians test preliminary versions of a system or systems that have not been completely debugged. If this happened, it would be extremely hard to engage them for another round of testing. This may sound like doing evaluations is impossible, but the problem can be managed and overcome with modern software development approaches. For example, if the developers use a spiral approach as their life cycle model, the researcher can test the first versions of the system with other less constrained users, for example, graduate students in healthcare, to flush out obvious problems. These proxy users can be primed to act as the intended user. Alternatively, if there are several modules that can be tested separately, the evaluations can be made as efficient as possible so that intended users can partake from the start. For example, algorithms can sometimes be tested individually by showing their outcome on a piece of paper or by email.

In addition to the practical problems related to time constraints, there are also additional, fundamental obstacles that make evaluating information systems difficult in a healthcare setting. If the intended user group consists of patients, other difficulties will surface. It will not always be easy to find access to patients and encourage them to participate in a study. Many patients will be too ill or too stressed to participate. Their main concern is becoming healthy again, and for many there is no motivation left to evaluate information systems and their impact. However, others will welcome an opportunity 'to make things better' for patients like them. Similar to studies with clinicians, the information system should be relevant to the patients. The researcher encounters the patients when they are most vulnerable. It is therefore crucial that one pays special attention to the treatment of the people, their information and how to keep results anonymous, ensuring informed consent of the patients who agreed to participate while making certain that one does not endanger therapy or negatively influence their outcomes.

Study Environment

To increase the external validity of evaluation studies, it is beneficial to test the information system in the field instead of in a laboratory environment and to use live data. Especially later in the developmental life cycle of information systems, when the system is more complete and would benefit from being tested as such, it becomes increasingly difficult to properly evaluate the system in a laboratory environment.

A good approach is to customize the type of testing being done to the development phase of the product. In early stages, when developing and fine-tuning algorithms, it may be best to use historical data that is offline. The output can then conveniently be combined and prepared in an efficient manner for offline evaluation.

For example, when developing a biomedical search engine, the matching algorithm needs to be evaluated. This can be done by testing a different version against a collection of documents. The matched documents can be presented to researchers for evaluation, for example, by having them score each abstract on a Likert scale for relevance. Similarly, the interface of an information system can often be tested very early in the development life cycle. Evaluating interfaces also is a good approach to getting very early feedback on the product. It helps make visible to the user what the system's capabilities and limitations will be, often leading to suggestions for change or improvements. Again, the interface should not be connected to the live data but should show representative data, either historic or simulated. Once the product is more complete, it becomes increasingly important to test it in a realistic environment. Testing in a real environment adds several layers of complexity because of complications related to the focus on safety in medicine. Precautions are then needed to ensure that no ongoing healthcare activities are influenced unduly.

Use of Live Data

The best evaluations will use data that is as realistic as possible and will work with users who are as representative as possible. Working with real data and actual patients and clinicians is the best. Again, caution is needed. Medicine is a safety first discipline. New systems should provide benefits and do no harm. Taking a step-by-step approach, where individual components of a system are first systemically tested in safe environments, e.g., by not impacting actual clinical decisions or patients, is therefore best. Once the system components have been tested, shown at a minimum to do no harm and preferably provide a benefit, more complete versions of a system can be tested in increasingly real settings.

The researcher conducting the evaluation should avoid influencing the ongoing decision process of the clinicians until the new system has been shown to be superior to the system that is in place. This restriction may make it seem impossible to conduct studies in a realistic setting, but it is not. For example, consider a decision support system that is intended to be used by practicing pediatricians. The system provides probabilities for the success of several therapies with past, similar cases. Assume the developers have completed their work and the decision support system is ready for testing with real data. There are two very good options for the researchers: working with live data but not the associated clinicians or working with historical but complete data.

When working with live data, it is possible to avoid problems by using the real data in real time but not involving the treating clinicians. For example, the researchers can show the results of the decision support system to pediatricians from a different hospital who are not on the case. With modern telemedicine techniques, this is quite doable.

Alternatively, working with historical data can be very valuable, realistic and more practical. Today's existence of logged data makes many evaluations possible without affecting safety and introducing breaches of privacy. Logs can be de-identified if necessary and allow early and valuable testing of systems even without involvement of clinicians. Such data logs can be used to test the functionality, efficiency and range of an information system. Can the system handle all different cases encountered in the logs and does it do so in an efficient manner? Such early testing will help uncover problems and will optimize the use of experts' time in later evaluations. By using logs, the data and the system outcomes can be compared to the decisions made by the clinicians. For example, when a new system is being developed, this data can be fed to the new system and its outcome compared to the logged outcome. Developers can use this comparison to report on results or have clinicians look at the comparisons to evaluate the differences between system and expert outcomes. Logs also can be used for more classical user studies. For example, a study can be designed to compare the treatments pediatricians would provide with and without your system. Because historical, closed cases are used, there is no danger this process will affect the actual, ongoing treatment.

HIPAA

In 1996, the Administrative Simplification provision of the Health Insurance Portability and Accountability Act (HIPAA) came into effect. While a complete discussion of HIPAA is beyond the scope of this book, a basic understanding of its effects on research is necessary for U.S. based researchers and those collaborating with U.S. based researchers. The goal of HIPAA is to protect healthcare insurance coverage for workers (part 1) and to mandate an electronic standard of information transactions to improve the administrative efficiency of healthcare transactions (part 2). This second part also addresses the protection of data and privacy issues.

The Privacy Rule issued by the Department of Health and Human Services came into effect in 2003. It protects the use and disclosure of identifiable information held by covered entities. This information also is known as protected health information (PHI). The covered entities comprise the healthcare providers, the healthcare clearing houses and others providing healthcare operations. Health information refers to information in any form that relates to the past, present and future physical and mental health conditions of a person. Protected health information refers to that health information that is individually identifiable and that is created or received by a covered entity. HIPAA was not intended to interfere with treatment or payment of healthcare operations. However, the Privacy Rule was intended as a protection of information in electronic format since it was seen as very easy to distribute and then be used for other than intended purposes. The restrictions are therefore on use of the data for operations other than treatment. This protection affects researchers' access to the data.

Simply put, under HIPAA, *permission is needed by the covered entities to disclose data*. Since in research many groups often share data, not only between researchers but also with review or data monitoring boards, the HIPAA Privacy Rule has enormous impact. Further, there are additional FDA regulations and the Common Rule which are different from HIPAA's Privacy Rules. Complicating matters, HIPAA also needs to be integrated with state and federal laws. The Privacy Rules provides a "floor" of protection. They override more lenient rules when they exist. Violations of the rules may lead to civil and criminal penalties.

Much data is available in medical format that could be used for research and faster and better medical treatments but that cannot currently be used for this purpose. Anderson and Schonfeld [46] show how using existing data could benefit development of treatments without needing further subject recruitment. Unfortunately, the informed consent forms used for these earlier studies are often problematic and do not include data sharing with a pharmaceutical or medical device company. As a result, that data and information cannot be shared and cannot be used in evaluations.

References

1. Murphy TE (2009) Requirements form the foundation of software quality. Research report, G00165755
2. Gonzales CK (2010) Eliciting user requirements using appreciative inquiry. Ph.D., Claremont Graduate University
3. Baroudi JJ, Olson MH, Ives B (1986) An empirical study of the impact of user involvement on system usage and information satisfaction. Commun ACM 29(3):232–238
4. Schneider GM, Martin J, Tsai WT (1992) An experimental study of fault detection in user requirements documents. ACM Trans Software Eng Methodol (TOSEM) 1(2):188–204. doi:10.1145/128894.128897
5. Westland JC (2002) The Cost of Errors in Software Development: Evidence from Industry. The Hournal of Systems and Software, 62, 1–9
6. Friedman CP, Wyatt JC (2000) Evaluation methods in medical informatics. Springer-Verlag, New York
7. Brender J (2006) Handbook of evaluation methods for health informatics (trans: Carlander L). Elsevier Inc, San Diego
8. Kaplan B (2001) Evaluating informatics applications — clinical decision support systems literature review. Int J Med Inform 64:15–37
9. Tesh EM, Holditch-Davis D (1997) HOME inventory and NCATS: relation to mother and child behaviors during naturalistic observations. Home observation for measurement of the environment. Nursing Child Assessment Teaching Scale. Res Nurs Health 20(4):295–307
10. Lambrechts G, Noortgate WVD, Eeman L, Maes B (2010) Staff reactions to challenging behaviour: an observation study. Res Dev Disabil 31:525–535
11. Campos B, Graesch AP, Repetti R, Bradbury T, Ochs E (2009) Opportunity for interaction? A naturalistic observation study of dual-earner families after work and school. J Fam Psychol 23(6):798–807
12. Kaplan B (2001) Evaluating informatics applications – some alternative approaches: theory, social interactionism, and call for methodological pluralism. Int J Med Inform 64:39–56
13. Rosson MB, Carroll JM (2002) Usability engineering: scenario-based development of human-computer interaction. Interactive technologies. Morgan Kaufman Publishers, San Francisco
14. Purkis ME (1999) Embracing technology: an exploration of the effects of writing nursing. Nurs Inq 6(3):147–156
15. Stringer ET (1999) Action research. SAGE Publications Inc, Thousand Oaks
16. Boursnell M, Prosser S (2010) Increasing identification of domestic violence in emergency departments: a collaborative contribution to increasing the quality of practice of emergency nurses. Contemp Nurse 35(12):7

17. Borg M, Karlsson B, Kim HS (2010) Double helix of research and practice - developing a practice model for crisis resolution and home treatment through participatory action research. Int J Qualitative Stud Health Well-being 5. doi: 10.3402/qhw.v5i1.4647

18. Butera-Prinzi F, Charles N, Heine K, Rutherford B, Lattin D (2010) Family-to-family link up program: a community-based initiative supporting families caring for someone with an acquired brain injury. NeuroRehabilitation 27:31–47

19. Davison R, Vogel D (2007) Group support systems in Hong Kong: an action research project. In: Galliers RD, Markus ML, Newell S (eds) Exploring information systems research approaches: readings and reflections. Routledge, New York, pp 33–46

20. Delobelle P, Onya H, Langa C, Mashamba J, Depoorter AM (2010) Advances in health promotion in Africa: promoting health through hospitals. Global Health Promot 17:33–36. doi:10.1177/1757975910363929

21. Rust J, Golombok S (2009) Modern psychometrics: the science of psychological assessment, 3rd edn. Routledge, London

22. Magnusson D (1966) Test theory. Addison-Wesley Publishing Company, Reading

23. Drenth PJD, Sijtsma K (1990) Testtheorie: Inleiding in de Theorie van de Psychologische Test en zijn Toepassingen. Bohn Stafleu Van Loghum, Houten/Antwerpen

24. de Ayala RJ (2009) The theory and practice of item response theory. Methodology in the social sciences. The Guilford Press, New York

25. Rushton P, Miller W, Lee KR, Eng J, Yip J (2011) Development and Content Validation of the Wheelchair Use Confidence Scale: A Mixed-Methods Study. Disability and Rehabilitation Assistive Technology, 6 (1), 57–66

26. Fischer B, Nakamura N, Ialomiteanu A, Boak A, Rehm J (2010) Assessing the prevalence of nonmedical prescription opioid use in the general Canadian population: methodological issues and questions. La Revue Canadienne De Psychiatrie 55(9):606–609

27. Jaussent S, Labarère J, Boyer J, François P (2004) Psychometric characteristics of questionnaires designed to assess the knowledge, perceptions and practices of health care professionals with regards to alcoholic patients [translation: article in French]. Encephale 30(5):437–446

28. Palmirotta R, Savonarola A, Ludovici G, Donati P, Cavaliere F, De Marchis M, Ferroni P, Guadagni F (2010) Association between Birt Hogg Dube syndrome and cancer predisposition. Anticancer Res 30(3):751–757

29. Ajzen I (1991) The theory of planned behavior. Organ Behav Hum Decis Process 50:179–211

30. Davis FD (1989) Perceived usefulness, perceived ease of use, and user acceptance of information technology. MIS Q 13(3):319–339

31. Hu PJ-H, Sheng ORL, Chau PY, Tam K-Y, Fung H (1999) Investigation physician acceptance of telemedicine technology: a survey study in Hong Kong. In: 32nd Hawaii International Conference on System Sciences, 1999

32. Hu PJ-H, Chau PYK, Sheng ORL (2000) Investigation of factors affecting healthcare organization's adoption of telemedicine technology. In: 33rd Hawaii international conference on system sciences, 2000

33. Rawstorne P, Jayasuriya R, Caputi P (2000) Issues in predicting and explaining usage behaviors with the technology acceptance model and the theory of planned behavior when usage is mandatory. In: International conference on information systems, Brisbane, Australia, 2000, pp 35–44

34. Honeth L, Bexelius C, Eriksson M, Sandin S, Litton J, Rosenhall U, Nyrén O, Bagger-Sjöbäck D (2010) An Internet-based hearing test for simple audiometry in nonclinical settings: preliminary validation and proof of principle. Otol Neurotol 31(5):708–714

35. Ives B, Olson MH, Baroudi JJ (1983) The measurement of user information satisfaction. Commun ACM 26(10):785–793

36. Chinman M, Young AS, Schell T, Hassell J, Mintz J (2004) Computer-assisted self-assessment in persons with severe mental illness. J Clin Psychiatry 65(10):1343–1351

37. Sunaert P, Bastiaens H, Nobels F, Feyen L, Verbeke G, Vermeire E, Maeseneer JD, Willems S, Sutter AD (2010) Effectiveness of the introduction of a chronic care model-based program for type 2 diabetes in Belgium. BMC Health Serv Res. doi:10.1186/1472-6963-10-207
38. Sunaert P, Bastiaens H, Feyen L, Snauwaert B, Nobels F, Wens J, Vermeire E, Royen PV, Maeseneer JD, Sutter AD, Willems S (2009) Implementation of a program for type 2 diabetes based on the chronic care model in a hospital-centered health care system: "the Belgian experience". BMC Health Services Research 9 (152). doi:10.1186/1472-6963-9-152
39. Herz EJ, Goldberg WA, Reis JS (1984) Family life education for young adolescents: a quasi-experiment. J Youth Adolesc 13(4):309–327
40. Glynn S, Randolph E, Garrick T, Lui A (2010) A proof of concept trial of an online psychoeducational program for relatives of both veterans and civilians living with schizophrenia. Psychiatr Rehabil J 33(4):278–287
41. Kröncke K (2010) Computer-based learning versus practical course in pre-clinical education: acceptance and knowledge retention. Med Teach 32(5):408–413
42. Kirk RE (1995) Experimental design: procedures for the behavioral sciences, 3rd edn. Brooks/Cole Publishing Company, Pacific Grove
43. Timm NH (2002) Applied multivariate analysis. Springer, New York
44. Everitt BS, Pickles A (2004) Statistical aspects of the design and analysis of clinical trials, Revisedth edn. Imperial College Press, London
45. Ammenwertha E, Gräber S, Herrmann G, Bürkle T, König J (2003) Evaluation of health information systems—problems and challenges. Int J Med Inform 71:125–135
46. Anderson JR, Schonfeld TL (2009) Data-sharing dilemmas: allowing pharmaceutical company access to research data. IRB: Ethics Hum Res 31(3):17–19

Variables

2

Chapter Summary

The previous chapter discussed how a clearly defined goal helps the researcher or developer choose the type of study to perform. In this and the following chapter, it is assumed that an experiment, referred to as a user study, is to be executed. Different names are used to describe such studies depending on the discipline. For example, experiments, as they are called in psychology, are more often called user studies in informatics or randomized clinical trials in medicine. Regardless of the name used, the design of the study will influence whether any interesting results are found and the degree to which these results can be trusted and generalized beyond the study.

This chapter describes the different types of variables that one needs to understand and define when conducting a user study. The independent variable is the treatment or the intervention. In informatics, this is usually the new system or algorithm that needs to be evaluated. It is compared against one or more other conditions, systems or algorithms. The dependent variable is the outcome or the result that is important to the users, developers or researchers. In informatics, it is often an improvement in processes or decisions that can be attributed to the new system or algorithm. How these two types of variables are defined and measured will affect the trustworthiness of the study and also how well the results can be generalized to other situations. Confounded variables, nuisance variables and bias all affect the relationship between independent and dependent variables. By controlling these additional variables and choosing the best design, the researcher can ensure the best possible, honest results. A poor design can lead to spurious conclusions, but more often it will lead to missing existing effects and a waste of time, money and effort.

G. Leroy, *Designing User Studies in Informatics*, Health Informatics,
DOI 10.1007/978-0-85729-622-1_2, © Springer-Verlag London Limited 2011

Independent Variables

The term *independent variable* means the same as *treatment* or *intervention* [1] and signifies a "causal event that is under investigation" [2]. The independent variable, manipulated by the researcher, describes what is expected to influence the outcomes. A treatment is a specific condition of this independent variable. The goal of a user study is to compare the outcomes for different treatments. The independent variable is connected to the dependent variable, which measures the outcome, by means of the hypotheses [3]. A simple hypothesis is a prediction of a causal effect of the independent variable on the dependent variable: depending on the condition of the independent variable a different outcome is predicted for the dependent variable.

A user study can have one or more than one independent variables and, in this case, each variable represents a treatment that can be controlled and systematically manipulated by the researcher. Studies with more than one independent variable are more complex to execute, analyze and interpret. The number of variables also affects the number of participants that need to be found for the study. Usually, more independent variables will mean that more subjects are needed. However, in some cases subjects can participate in multiple conditions.

In medical informatics, many studies will evaluate the impact of one independent variable only. This independent variable includes a new or improved information system that is to be compared with other, older approaches. For example, assume a researcher has designed a persuasive text messaging system that uses text messaging to encourage obese people to lose weight. The system sends messages a few times a day about possible activities that are suitable given the day of the week and the weather forecast. The goal is to help people lose weight by encouraging them to engage in physical activity. The study will test whether the persuasive messaging system is more effective than, for example, meetings with a dietician. However, it is possible to consider other independent variables. In this example, the researchers suspect that the system will be more suitable for younger users because most already love using their mobile phone. So the researchers also want to compare older and younger people, which can be defined as a second independent variable.

Types of Variables

The independent variables can be of different types, and these different types can be present in the same study. Understanding the types will help the researcher choose the levels to be used in the study. *Qualitative independent variables* describe different kinds of treatments. For example, a qualitative independent variable called "System Availability" could have two conditions: the presence (condition 1) or absence (condition 2) of the information system. Such a qualitative comparison also could be made between two types of systems, or between an information system and behavioral therapy, among others. In all these examples, there are two or more conditions for one independent variable. For the weight loss messenger system described above, it would be possible to compare weight loss of people who use

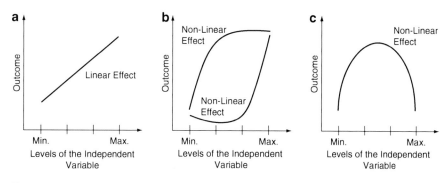

Fig. 2.1 Example effects

the system versus people who work with a dietician. In many cases, the current situation, and this can consist of an existing information system or a non-computer information system, serves as a baseline. For example, Gorini et al. [4] compare three conditions for treating generalized anxiety disorder: one condition consists of using virtual reality via a mobile phone with biofeedback, a second condition consists of the virtual reality via a mobile phone but without biofeedback and a third condition consists of no intervention.

Quantitative independent variables compare different amounts of a given treatment. For example, one could compare sending one message per day with sending one message during every daytime hour. When using a quantitative independent variable, it is important to carefully consider which levels to use. Especially when conducting an initial evaluation of a system, it is best to evaluate levels taken from a wide enough range so that the results will show as much of the impact as possible. If possible, include two extremes and at least one, but better two, levels in between. This will improve understanding the effect of the intervention.

For example, as shown in Fig. 2.1a, a linear effect may be present where the outcome is directly proportional to the input. Having only two levels will make it hard to show the type of relationship that exists. Figures 2.1b and 2.1c show other relationships where it is advantageous to have multiple levels of the independent variable. Figure 2.1b shows a relationship where the extremes are not the best values and where the effect of the independent variable levels off. Often this happens when the intermediate levels represent a more balanced treatment approach. Similarly, Fig. 2.1c shows how the extreme conditions do not present the best outcome. Worse, no effect at all would be noticeable if only the extremes were measured. With new systems, the extreme situation may still be unknown and a poorly designed study will lead to the conclusion that there is no effect, while the study only failed to measure it.

Use common sense when deciding on the levels of the independent variable. Consider theoretical reasons as well as ethical and practical limitations. Consider the following treatment levels of the text messaging system: the lower extreme value, the minimum, could be 1 message per day; the highest level, the maximum, could be 32 messages or 1 message every 30 min during the day. One message a day may have no effect at all, while receiving a message every 30 min may be annoying and have adverse effects, such as people turning off their phones so they do not receive any more messages.

Note about Random Assignment

It is important to remember that random assignment of subjects to the experimental conditions is what makes a study a true experiment. By randomly assigning subjects to conditions, one can avoid systematic distortion of the results. A note of caution is needed however. Even though random assignment is critical to discover causal relations, it may introduce a new bias, especially in medicine. With many studies, especially clinical trials, patients or consumers will have a preference for a certain treatment; they usually prefer to receive the new treatment. For some patients, it is their last hope. Random selection does not take this preference into account, and this may influence enrolment, sample representativeness, attrition, adherence or compliance, and outcomes [5]. For example, only patients who are willing to be part of a placebo condition may participate, or patients may drop out when they suspect they are not receiving the new treatment.

Dependent Variables

A *dependent variable* is also called an *outcome* or *response variable* [1, 6] and represents the outcome of a treatment. The dependent variable should be chosen so that one can make a conclusion about the treatment in relation to the professed goal. It is expected that this dependent variable will show different outcomes for the different experimental conditions. If the goal is to develop an information system that helps people with weight loss, the dependent variable should reflect this goal and allow the researchers to draw conclusions about losing weight with help from the information system that is being evaluated. For example, the weight lost after 1 month could be the dependent variable. For the persuasive text messaging system described above, it is expected and hypothesized that participants will lose more weight with the text messaging system than without.

A good evaluation will have complementary measures to assess the impact of a treatment. When the outcomes of complementary measures point in the same direction, for example, that a system is user friendly, this provides a much stronger evaluation and the researcher can be much more confident about the conclusion. Moreover, such additional measures often are useful to help explain unexpected results of using the system. Keep in mind that each analysis will evaluate the impact of the conditions, the independent variable, on one outcome measure, the dependent variable, at a time.

When choosing a set of evaluation metrics, it is important to include existing metrics decision makers are already familiar with when possible. Regardless whether the decision makers are the future users, the buyers of the software or fellow researchers, metrics used for many years or in many evaluations are more likely to be well understood and accepted as part of the decision making process. Naturally, relying solely on metrics that have been used historically is unwise. Evaluations should include the metrics that are most relevant to the study. For example, if one designed a system for online appointment scheduling, the clinic where the system will be tested will most probably already keep track of the number of people who do not show up for appointments. Obviously, they will be interested in seeing the effects of the system on such a well known metric. In addition, it may be quite reasonable to measure the number of changes in appointments and the associated costs. A new system may not only affect no-shows but also the time needed for rescheduling existing appointments.

Below, a general approach to categorizing variables and measures is described. This is followed by a list of commonly used metrics. The metrics to be used are often determined by the field of study, the environment or the decision makers; however, it is important to remember that the choice of the metric also will affect the power of the study or how sensitive it is. Some metrics are better than others to show a significant effect even when used on the same dataset. For example, when an ordered list is being evaluated, rank order metrics, which take the order into account, show a higher effect size than all-or-none metrics, where only the presence of the correct answer counts [7].

Types of Variables

There is a broad choice of possible dependent variables. They have different advantages and disadvantages, and their popularity depends on the field of study. One way of looking at the types of variables is to categorize them according to the aspect of the information that is being evaluated. Goodman and Ahn [8] list five categories of measures: technical properties; safety; efficacy and efficiency; economic attributes or impacts; and legal, social, ethical or political impacts. Below are examples of many measurements that belong to the first three categories. The last two are beyond the scope of this book.

The development phase of a project affects the choice of dependent variable. There are several outcome measures that are suitable for use in multiple phases of the system's life cycle stage. However, there are other outcome measures that are particularly suited to early or late development phases. As Kushniruk and Patel [9] point out, usability evaluations are especially useful during the formative phases of the software. Waiting until the final development stages or implementation to test usability is not a good idea. Problems with the interface and expected interactions between the system and users need to be caught early. With current software toolkits, user interfaces can be prototyped very early in the development cycle and tested with a variety of measures. During explorative, early phases of development, measures such as relevance, completeness of results, feasibility and risk will take center stage. Many other measures, such as cost savings or improved decision making, are usually better suited for later stages, when the system has reached maturity.

Once it has been decided what the dependent variable will be, it is necessary to choose a metric. Metrics are the measurement tools. For example, an already existing, validated survey instrument could be used to measure user preference. Another example is the use of a formula to calculate precision or recall. The metrics provide the concrete value for the chosen measure [10]. It is best to have a combination of measures for a study to have a balanced evaluation. The simplest and most straightforward approach is to use *single* or *base metrics*. However, sometimes *derived* or *composite metrics* are needed. This distinction also is referred to as *base* versus *synthetic metrics* [11].

For example, to determine user friendliness, one measure could be the subjective evaluation of system's user friendliness with a survey. However, in most studies, participants will be required to complete a task that allows additional metrics to be measured. For example, a complementary metric could be a count of the number of errors made when working on the tasks, which would capture objectively how user friendly the system was. When working with tasks, it is important that they are representative of the final intended usage of the system. Otherwise, the metrics will be irrelevant. For example, if a clinician is required to evaluate only one x-ray per half hour, the speed of loading the x-ray on the screen will not be that important. It should not matter whether it loads in 500 ms or in 1 s and a dependent variable measuring load time would be pointless in this case. However, when evaluating a decision support system where a few thousand images are loaded and clustered for a clinician to review, the time it takes to load them will be extremely important.

For study designers who have complete discretion over the choice of dependent variables, a good trio to consider is: effectiveness, efficiency and satisfaction. *Effectiveness* measures whether the information system does what it is supposed to do. Examples are the number of errors, counts of (relevant) events, precision, recall, and false positives and false negatives, among others. *Efficiency* measures whether the information system does its job in a suitable manner. Examples are whether tasks were completed, time taken to complete the task, run time and memory requirements, among others. An alternative view on these two measures is outcome versus performance measures. *Outcome measures* are used to evaluate the results of applying the information system, similar to effectiveness measures, while *performance measures* are used to evaluate the process itself, similar to efficiency measures. *Satisfaction measures* are more subjective and relate to the users' perception of a system. Example measures range from simple questions such as "Which system do you prefer?" (when comparing systems) to multi-item validated questionnaires.

Common Information Retrieval Measures

Precision, Recall and the F-measure are three outcomes that are among the most frequently used in information systems evaluations. Precision and recall are individual measures, while the F-measure is a composite value, providing a balanced number that combines both precision and recall. They are particularly popular in the evaluation of information retrieval systems. Yousefi-Nooraie et al. [12] use precision and recall to compare three different PubMed search filters that are meant to help answer clinical questions. Kullo et al. [13] use precision and recall to evaluate algorithms that extract information from electronic medical records for use in genome-wide association studies.

Precision refers to how accurate a result set is. For example, when testing a search engine, precision indicates how many of the results returned in response to a query are relevant (see Eq. 2.1). *Recall*, on the other hand, refers to how much of the relevant information is contained in the result set (see Eq. 2.2). With a search engine evaluation, recall refers to the number of relevant items in the results set compared to all possible relevant items. Usually, a trade-off can be observed between precision and recall. When a system is tuned to be more precise, the recall goes down. When a system is tuned for higher recall, the precision goes down. Because of this trade-off, it is often difficult to compare information systems and the F-measure is sometimes preferred because it combines both measures (see Eq. 2.3).

$$Precision = \frac{\# \, retrieved \, and \, relevant \, items}{\# \, retrieved \, items} \tag{2.1}$$

$$Recall = \frac{\# \, retrieved \, and \, relevant \, items}{\# \, relevant \, items} \tag{2.2}$$

$$F - measure = 2 * \frac{Precision * Recall}{Precision + Recall} \tag{2.3}$$

As noted above, the *F-measure* is a weighted average of precision and recall. In the best possible scenario, when both precision and recall are perfect, the F-measure's value is 1. In the worst possible scenario, when precision or recall is 0, the F-measure's value is 0. For example, assume there is a set of records and a subset of those is considered to be relevant to an information request. A search engine has been constructed to retrieve those relevant records from the entire set with a given query. When the query is executed, the search engine retrieves all relevant documents and no others. In this best case, precision is 100% and recall is 100%, resulting in an F-measure of 1. However, had the search engine retrieved no relevant documents, precision and subsequently the F-measure's value would be 0.

Classification Measures

Many algorithms and information systems are developed with the intent to automatically categorize or label people, records or other data items. They perform a type of prediction called classification. Based on a set of rules, a label is automatically assigned to each data point. The rules can be acquired with machine learning algorithms, based on codified expert knowledge or with statistical calculations.

There may be different kinds of labels that can be assigned. For example, algorithms can be trained to distinguish between two classes for brain images displaying a mass and label them as either benign growths or tumors.

Evaluating such a system entails finding out whether the label was assigned correctly. Several measures can be used for this. In the informatics community, *accuracy* is the most common measure used to evaluate the correctness of classification. Measuring accuracy requires that a gold standard is available to compare the algorithm outcome against the correct solution. Accuracy then refers to the percentage of items correctly classified in an entire set as compared against the gold standard (see Eq. 2.4). For example, if there is a set of mammograms with a subset known to display a tumor, then accuracy of an algorithm would be evaluated by calculating how many mammograms were correctly classified as containing a tumor or not. In medical informatics, accuracy is described using four more specific metrics: True Positives (TP), True Negatives (TN), False Positives (FP) and False Negatives (FN). In addition, other derived measures are commonly used that form combinations of these four, namely specificity and sensitivity. However, this nomenclature is useful when only two classes are being distinguished. When there are more classes, a confusion matrix is a better choice. Each of these measures is described in detail below.

$$Accuracy = \frac{TP + TN}{TP + TN + FP + FN} \tag{2.4}$$

The *True Positive, True Negative, False Positive* and *False Negative* classification can be used with a gold standard for evaluating system, algorithm and even expert classifications. For example, assume a neural network has been trained to distinguish between cancerous and normal tissue on images displaying masses. After training the algorithm, it is evaluated using a dataset for which the correct outcome is known. If such an algorithm classified an image as showing cancerous tissue, this is considered a True Positive (see Eq. 2.5) when that is a correct decision. However, if the image did not show cancerous tissue, the algorithm would be wrong and this would be called a False Positive (see Eq. 2.7). Similarly, if the algorithm correctly classified an image as not showing cancerous tissue, this is called a True Negative (see Eq. 2.6) if this was the correct decision. Again, if the tissue had been cancerous after all, then the algorithm was wrong and the decision would be called a False Negative (see Eq. 2.8). While the terms TP, TN, FP and FN are most commonly used in medicine, there are synonymous terms which are more commonly used in psychology: Hit instead of TP, Correct Rejection instead of TN, False Alarm instead of FP and Miss instead of FN. Table 2.1 shows an overview of this classification.

$$True\ Positive\ (Hit) = an\ instance\ correctly\ labeled\ as \tag{2.5}$$
$$belonging\ to\ a\ group$$

$$True\ Negative\ (Correct\ Rejection) = an\ instance\ correctly\ labeled \tag{2.6}$$
$$as\ not\ belonging\ to\ a\ group$$

Table 2.1 Demonstration of classification measures for two classes

Actual outcome	System predicted outcome		Total
	Diabetes	No diabetes	
Diabetes	TP	FN	
No diabetes	FP	TN	
Total			

$$False\ Positive\ (False\ Alarm) = an\ instance\ incorrectly\ labeled \quad (2.7)$$
$$as\ belonging\ to\ a\ group$$

$$False\ Negative\ (Miss) = an\ instance\ incorrectly\ labeled\ as\ not \quad (2.8)$$
$$belonging\ to\ a\ group$$

As noted above, in medical informatics the TP, TN, FP and FN are also combined into two additional, derived metrics. *Sensitivity* (see Eq. 2.9), also called the *detection rate*, refers to how well positive instances can be detected. *Specificity* (see Eq. 2.10) is a reference to how correctly that decision is made; in other words, how often the test correctly detects cancerous tissue.

$$Sensitivity = \frac{TP}{TP + FN} \quad (2.9)$$

$$Specificity = \frac{TN}{FP + TN} \quad (2.10)$$

In medicine, these specific measures help evaluate systems and tests relative to their intended use. For examples, for a serious and life-threatening disease such as HIV, a diagnosis of that disease is devastating, stressful and will lead to a battery of follow-up tests and treatments. Therefore it is essential that the specificity is high to avoid unnecessary stress and treatment. On the other hand, missing such a serious disease is disastrous too, and so the test should be sensitive enough. In addition to differences based on the seriousness of the disease, the timing of diagnosis also plays a role. Sometimes, clinicians want to use tests with high sensitivity for screening or early detection and follow up with tests with high specificity to confirm a diagnosis. In addition to providing such evaluations, it is also common to compare new tests with existing tests for sensitivity and specificity, as was done, for example, for a genetic algorithm/support vector machine combined algorithm to find protein-protein interactions [14], scoring systems to predict blood stream infection in patients [15] or a search engine to search and identify cancer cases in pathology reports [16].

When there are only two classes possible, the TP, TN, FP, FN notation is sufficient. However, in machine learning algorithm evaluations, a different notation is used that can easily be extended to more than two classes: a *confusion matrix* or *contingency table*. A confusion matrix is a better tool to evaluate the results with

Table 2.2 Demonstration of classification measures for four classes

	System predicted outcome				
Actual outcome	Type 1 diabetes	Type 2 diabetes	Gestational diabetes	No diabetes	Total
Type 1 diabetes	X1	a	b	c	Y1
Type 2 diabetes	d	X2	e	f	Y2
Gestational diabetes	g	h	X3	i	Y3
No diabetes	j	k	l	X4	Y4
Total	Z1	Z2	Z3	Z4	

multiple classes. It can be seen as the extension of the foursome discussed above adjusted to multiple outcome classes. A confusion matrix provides accuracy numbers per class and also provides details on how errors are classified. When evaluating systems or algorithms, these measures provide an indication of how well algorithms can be used to complete tasks that are often labor intensive and boring for humans. It should be noted that the human classification process itself is seldom error free.

For example, assume a system has been trained to predict who will get diabetes based on data in electronic medical records. It is possible to have any of three types of diabetes or to have no diabetes at all. After running the classification algorithms on the training data (training the model), the outcome is evaluated using test data. The algorithm classification of this test data is compared against the actual outcome. A confusion matrix can provide a detailed evaluation. For example, if very many errors are made in classifying instances as gestational diabetes, one of the conditions, this would not be clear from reporting true positives and true negative but it would be apparent in the confusion matrix.

Table 2.2 shows how such an evaluation looks for a classification with four possible outcomes. The true positives in the case of four labels can be found on the diagonal (X1, X2, X3, X4). The other numbers in the matrix (a-l) show the errors and provide details of how the records are classified incorrectly. For example, there are *a* records classified as belonging to people with Type 2 diabetes that should have been diagnosed with Type 1 diabetes. The totals (Y1, Y2, Y3, Y4 and Z1, Z2, Z3, Z4) provide rates for each specific class. For example, Z1 records were predicted to belong to people with Type 1 diabetes; X1 of these were correct. And Y1 records belonged to people with Type 1 diabetes while the system predicted only X1 of these correctly.

N-Fold Cross-Validation

When the rules to classify or label instances, such as patients, images or records, are learned by algorithms without human intervention (machine learning), a dataset can be used multiple times. This is done by dividing the entire set into *n* subsets which are called folds. This is possible with machine learning algorithms because their memory can be erased from one dataset to another so that each evaluation can be seen as independent. With *n-fold cross-validation*, each data point is randomly assigned to one of *n* subsets. Once the dataset is divided, one set is set apart for

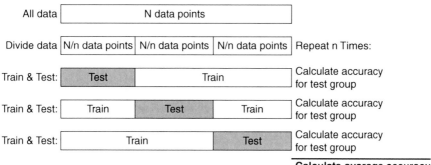

Fig. 2.2 N-fold cross-validation example (N = 3)

testing and the remaining $(n-1)$ sets are used for training the algorithm. Once training has been completed, the algorithm is tested on the set that was kept apart. The accuracy of the algorithm predictions is calculated for that test set. Note that the test set was not contained in the training data for the algorithm, and so this evaluation is for data that the algorithm will not have encountered during training. This process is repeated as many times as there are folds (n). The accuracy is then averaged over all folds. N-fold cross-validation cannot be used when rules are learned and encoded by a human because a person is unable to ignore the previous round of training and would be biased by previous interactions with the data.

As an example, Fig. 2.2 shows the process of evaluating a classification algorithm using 3-fold cross-validation $(n=3)$. Assume a dataset is available that contains N mammograms. Each mammogram shows a mass which is known to be benign or not based on a biopsy that was conducted. The entire dataset is labeled with the correct answer: benign or not benign. The algorithm is developed to read those images and learn whether the mass is benign or not. The goal is to use such an algorithm as a second opinion for new mammograms showing a mass. With 3-fold cross-validation, the dataset is split into three equal groups: each subset has one-third of the mammograms. Training of the classification model[1] and subsequent testing is repeated three times. The model is first trained using the combined data from two subsets and tested on a third. This provides the first accuracy measure. This process is completed three times. Each fold or subset serves as the test set once. The final accuracy is the average of the three accuracy numbers.

There are several advantages to this approach. First of all, the evaluation is repeated n times and does not depend on a single outcome. If each evaluation results in high accuracy scores, this is a good indication that the algorithm is stable. The test dataset may contain many examples the algorithm was not trained for and so the results would be worse than expected with other datasets. It is also possible that the test dataset contains mostly examples that the algorithm is highly trained for and

---

[1] Such training is done with supervised machine learning techniques also called classifiers. For example, a feedforward/backpropagation neural network (FF/BP), decision tree or other type of classifier could be used.

so the results will be better than expected with other datasets. To avoid reliance on one dataset, the common evaluation approach is to do n-fold cross-validation or *n* evaluations using the same dataset. In addition to a balanced evaluation, this approach is also useful for training the algorithm because it avoids over-fitting of the data.

The random assignment to n-folds may be adjusted to ensure that each subset is sufficiently representative of the entire dataset. This should be considered when there are classes in the dataset that appear very infrequently. If none of the examples belonging to this rare class was present in the training dataset, it would be impossible for the algorithm to learn its characteristics. For such datasets, stratified sampling would provide a more balanced approach of division into folds and would ensure that each subset has examples from each possible class.

For example, assume there is a dataset consisting of electronic health records (EHR) and researchers have developed an algorithm to predict which type of diabetes (if any) is associated with different characteristics. Each record in the dataset has a label associated with it indicating whether the person has diabetes and which type: Type 1 diabetes, Type 2 diabetes, gestational diabetes or no diabetes. This dataset is used to train the new algorithm to learn people's characteristics and if they are associated with diabetes. Since the number of people with gestational diabetes may be very small, the researchers should ensure that at least a few of these cases appear in each fold. Which ones will appear in a specific fold can be decided by random assignment to ensure that all records of women with gestational diabetes do not end up in one fold. If they were to end up in one fold, the algorithm would not be able to generalize information of this type in the evaluation. Software packages, e.g., Weka [17], usually include this option for evaluation and let the user choose the number of folds to be used.

Counts

Counts are a simple and often effective approach to evaluation. In many cases, several critical events can be counted that are indicative of the quality of a system. Some of these events are desired, while others need to be avoided. For example, with a decision support system, it is important to support correct decisions. In other cases, for example, a medical records system, it is important to reduce the amount of clicking and page visits needed to complete a record. Counting such events can contribute significantly to understanding why a system is accepted by users or not.

Sometimes, it will be necessary for the experimenter to observe the users' interactions with the system. However, be aware that few users will act in the same way when observed as when they are not. When people know they are being observed their behavior is not always completely natural. Luckily, counts often can be conducted by logging interactions with a system. For example, when conducting a study to evaluate a user interface it is possible to establish which links should or should not be followed because the assigned task and required outcome are known. In these cases, links followed in error can be tracked and they can be seen as indications that the interface is not intuitive.

Since counts are simple evaluation measures, they may not tell the entire story and it is best to complement them with other measures. The researcher also should consider how much emphasis should be put on these counts when explaining the study to the participants and when interpreting results. For example, with new software interfaces, many users will explore the new software and click many menus and options. This is not necessarily an error. If every click counts, the participants in the study should be aware of this so they focus on the task at hand without exploring.

Usability

Usability is an important characteristic of every information system. Today, an information system that could be considered perfect in all aspects but that was not usable or user friendly would not be considered acceptable. There are different approaches to measuring usability. A very popular approach in informatics is the use of survey based measures of usability. Validated surveys exist for this purpose. For example, the Software Usability Measurement Inventory (SUMI) developed by Kirakowski [18] contains 50 statements measuring five dimensions of usability: Efficiency, Affect, Helpfulness, Control and Learnability. Unfortunately, many researchers quickly put together a survey without taking any possible biases into account or without any validation. The conclusions that can be made using such an instrument are doubtful.

In addition to using surveys, usability also can be measured in an objective manner by counting events, counting errors or measuring task completion. Many different measures can be constructed in this manner. The more interesting measures compare different users on their training or task completion times. For example, when an information system is extremely usable, there should be little training time required. Some good examples of such systems can be found in museums where the goal is to have zero training time information systems. Visitors to the museum can walk up to a computer and use the information system without any training. Another good evaluation of usability is based on the comparison between novice and expert users. For example, REU or Relative User Efficiency (see Eq. 2.11), as described by Kirakoswki [11], is the time an ordinary user would need to complete a task compared to the time needed by an expert user:

$$RUE = \frac{Ordinary\ User\ Time}{Expert\ User\ Time} * 100 \tag{2.11}$$

User Satisfaction and Acceptance

User satisfaction and user acceptance are generally related to each other, and both factors are often measured with a onetime survey. However, often users need to be satisfied with a system in the short term before the system will be accepted in the long term. As a result, measuring acceptance becomes more meaningful when more time has passed for users to get acquainted with the system.

Almost every user study of information systems will contain a user satisfaction survey. Most of these surveys are filled out at the end of limited time interaction with the new system. Unfortunately, very few of these surveys have been validated. An exception is the Computer Usability Satisfaction Survey developed by Lewis [19]. It contains 19 items divided over 3 subscales: System Usefulness, Information Quality and Interface Quality. The 19 items are presented with a 7-point Likert scale ranging from "Strongly Agree" (score 1) to "Strongly disagree" (score 7), with a "Not Applicable" option outside the scale. The survey is fast and easy for study participants to complete [20, 21].

Many researchers and developers of information systems use their own surveys, but the usefulness, validity, objectivity and reliability of these is often questionable. It is very difficult to compose a survey that measures specific constructs. Wording of questions and answers will affect the results, biases will affect the results and many surveys will be incomplete or not measure what they intend to measure. It is therefore much better to use a survey that has been validated. This makes it possible to compare with other systems and be reasonably sure that the answers will be meaningful. Those researchers intending to develop their own survey should consult and learn the basics of psychometry, the field in psychology concerned with composing and conducting surveys. Evaluation of information systems is much more straightforward than psychological studies, since there deception is seldom necessary to measure constructs of interest. However, being knowledgeable on how to avoid biases, how to conduct a valid survey and how to avoid overlapping items measuring the same construct will improve any survey.

Processing Resources

Time and memory are two processing resources that are very suitable for evaluating individual algorithms. In algorithm development, there is a common trade-off between time and memory needed to complete a task. If all other factors are equal, a shorter processing time usually requires more memory, while using less memory will usually result in more processing time being needed.

A complexity analysis is a formal approach to evaluating an algorithm's runtime or memory usage in comparison to the input given to the algorithm. B*ig-O analysis* is a commonly used complexity analysis. It provides an evaluation of an algorithm independent of the specific computer or processor being used. This analysis is important since information systems may show very good evaluation results, but may be too complex to be used in a realistic setting. The "O" refers to "in the *O*rder of ..." [22]. The analysis is used to define the worst case or average case of an algorithm's hold on resources (time or memory) in relation to the given input (N). It is very useful when describing algorithms with varying performance. The analysis focuses on the loops in an algorithm and allows comparison of space or processing time in terms of order of magnitude.

For example, if the input datasets consist of N items, then an algorithm that runs in O(N) time is an algorithm that runs in linear time: the amount of time needed to complete is directly related to the number of input items. However, an algorithm that runs in $O(N^2)$ needs much more time to complete. It needs NxN or N^2 to complete processing a dataset with N input items. This analysis provides a simple measure that is expressed as an order of magnitude. For example, it does not matter whether the time increase was 6x or 200x times the input X, both would be noted as O(N). Similarly, if the algorithm requires $(x^2 + 10x)$ time for an input of X, it would be noted that the algorithm runs in $O(N^2)$. For a detailed description of how to conduct this analysis, the reader is referred to Nance and Naps [22] or other introductory computer science books covering algorithm and data structure analysis.

Although computer speed and memory have become a commodity for many simple applications, in medicine and biomedicine there are several applications where such analysis is essential, for example, visualization of protein folding or image analysis of moving organs. The analysis is essential in the development of many algorithms that will become part of sophisticated software packages. For example, Xiao et al. [23] describe the reduced complexity of such a new algorithm used in tomography, a technique used to reconstruct data for many types of medical scans. The algorithm complexity was reduced from $O(N^4)$ to $O(N^3logN)$.

Confounded Variables

Two variables are confounded when their effects cannot be separated from each other. When designing user studies, this problem is encountered when there is a variable other than the independent variable that may have caused the effect being studied. The variable causing the confounding reduces the internal validity of the study [24]: one cannot say for sure that the treatment, i.e., the independent variable, caused the effect. This variable changes with the experimental variable but was not intended to do so. As a result, the effect of the treatment cannot be attributed to the independent variable but may well have been caused by the other variable, the confounder. In some cases, confounded variables are difficult to avoid. Consider, for example, an experimenter effect. Most participants who voluntarily participate in user studies wish the researchers well and hope they succeed. If they know which condition the experimenters favor, they may evaluate it more positively.

To avoid having confounded variables, it is important to take possible bias into account, to make sure participants are assigned randomly to experimental conditions and to verify that the independent variable is the sole element that can be causing the effect. Consider the example of a weight loss support system that uses text messages and that is compared against another support system that does not use text messages. For practical reasons, the researchers may decide that it is easier to assign the text message condition to subjects who already possess a mobile phone because it makes it easier to run the study. Study participants without a mobile phone are assigned to the condition that does not use text messaging. With this design, it is very probable that the researchers have introduced confounded variables which make it impossible to conclude that any differences in weight loss between the two groups can be attributed to the text messaging system. For example, compared to participants who possess a mobile phone, participants without mobile phones may belong to a less affluent demographic group with a different lifestyle, different access to health information and a different attitude to healthy living.

Several approaches can be taken to avoid losing validity due to confounded variables. Naturally, the best approach is to design the experiment such that confounding variables are avoided. When this is not possible, other precautions can be taken that would allow the researcher to draw valid conclusions. First, one can use demographic data to measure possible confounding. When conducting a user study, it is useful to collect additional demographic data so that expected confounding can be objectively evaluated. Systematic differences in such variables between conditions would indicate confounding variables. However, if experimental groups do not differ on these measures, the study is strengthened. For example, when evaluating the weight loss support system, researchers could collect information about education levels, reading comprehension and even attitudes toward healthy living. They could then compare whether there are systematic differences between the experimental groups with regard to these variables.

A second approach to avoid making conclusions based on confounded variables is to include complementary outcome measures in the study. When such complementary measures are used, contradictions in their outcomes may be an indication that there are confounded variables. In studies with the elderly, the author and her students observed such confounding between the experimental condition, a new versus an old user interface, and an experimenter effect. Usability was evaluated with subjective and objective measures. The study participants mentioned they enjoyed their time working with the graduate students and wanted to help them graduate. This was clearly visible in the participants' survey ratings; it could be concluded that the participants *loved* the new system compared to the old system. However, the objective measures used did not show any benefit of the new system over the old.

A third approach is to improve the design to avoid possible confounding. With new information technology, such as telemedicine or virtual reality, many more options to improve study designs and avoid bias are available. For example, in studies where communication styles or other similar characteristics are correlated with other personal characteristics, there could be confounded variables. Mast et al. [25] evaluated the impact of gender versus the communication styles of physicians on patient satisfaction. In most cases, the communication style is very much related to gender. As a result, it is extremely difficult to pinpoint which of the two affects patients' satisfaction. Information technology helped disentangle these variables. Using a virtual physician, the researchers were able to control each variable independently and measure the effects on patient satisfaction. The results showed it was the caring style, not the gender, which affected satisfaction.

Finally, other designs and analyses can take potential confounding into account and even use it. Multivariate statistical analysis can be used to take the effect of confounded variables into account [1]. In other cases, some controlled confounding is sometimes integrated into the design to reduce the number of participants needed to complete a study. These complex study designs, which are more common in the behavioral sciences, are discussed, for example, in Chap. 13 of Kirk [2].

Bias Caused by Nuisance Variables

Nuisance variables are variables that add variation to the study outcome that is not due to the independent variables and that is of no interest to the experimenter. They introduce undesired variation that reduces the chance of detecting the systematic impact of the independent variable. Even if there is a true difference between the experimental conditions, it may be undetectable if there is too much variation unrelated to the experimental conditions. If this type of variation is unsystematic, it is called *noise*. When the variation is systematic, it is a called *bias* [2]. If this bias also coincides with the levels of the independent variable, then the independent variable and the bias are confounded variables. Blocking, which can be used to counter some bias, is explained in Chap. 5 (blocking one nuisance variable) and Chap. 6 (blocking multiple nuisance variables). Other countermeasures to such bias are discussed in Chap. 13.

For example, assume a researcher is interested in the effects of caffeine on alertness in executive MBA classes, which are usually held in the evenings. It has been decided that the independent variable will be the number of cups of coffee: 0, 1 or 5. The dependent variable is the alertness in class and will be measured with a self-administered survey. All students in the class have agreed to participate in the study. The researchers realized that some students may have had a big meal before attending class, while others may hold out until after class. So, a nuisance variable in this study consists of eating (or not) a big meal before going to class. This variable will affect the outcome because participants will be less alert after that big meal. Thus, this nuisance variable needs to be controlled, for example, by giving all students a big meal before class. Then, any change in the measured alertness cannot be attributed to whether or not a meal was eaten.

Bias is a well studied topic and there are several famous experiments demonstrating bias. Many types of bias have received their own names over the years because they commonly appear in studies. Learning about these different types of bias will help the researcher design a better experiment by countering them as much as possible. Controlling the nuisance variables and the bias will increase the validity of the experiment and also the chances of discovering a true effect.

Subject-Related Bias

One subject-related bias is the *good subject effect*. This effect is the result of study subjects who act in a certain way because they know they are participating in a study. There are three types of good subject effects. The first type is the effect that is most often associated with being a good subject, which involves some form of *altruism*. Such subjects are trying to give the researcher what he wants; they act in a way they believe is appropriate for the study and the treatment condition. There are two problems that result from this bias. The first is that the subjects do not behave naturally but act, i.e., they alter their behavior. The second is that the change in behavior is based on what the subjects believe or understand about the study. However, their understanding may be incomplete or wrong. With the emphasis on participants' satisfaction in many information systems' evaluations, this effect must be controlled. When the researcher is a doctoral student doing a dissertation study, subjects may be especially inclined to help the student with his research.

The second type of good subject effect is due to subjects who change their behavior as the result of a desire to comply with an *authority*. The subjects may feel that the researcher knows best. As a result, the study subjects may not feel qualified to argue, disagree or even voice an opinion. This is particularly true in medicine where the clinic staff is seen as the authority by patients, and so this effect may affect studies where patients or their caregivers are the subjects. In addition, there is also a clear hierarchy among the clinical staff members that may lead to the same type of bias and affect results in studies where the participants are clinical personnel.

Finally, a third type of good subject effect, the *look good effect* or the *evaluation apprehension effect*, is related to how the study subjects feel about themselves. Subjects who participate in experiments are often self-aware. They know they are being observed and they want to look good as a person. It is not clear how much this effect plays a role when evaluating software where behavior based measures, such as the number of errors made, are added to belief based measures, such as how good one feels or how much pain one feels. However, researchers should be aware of the effect and take it into consideration when forming conclusions.

Several studies have been done to evaluate and compare these biases. In the 1970s, a series of carefully controlled experiments was conducted to compare the different good subject effects [24, 26–28]. One of the goals of these studies was to tease apart the different origins of the good subject effect and discover the most influential reason. The evidence points mostly in the direction of a look good effect. When the look good and the altruism effect are competing factors, it seems that looking good becomes more important and is the main motivation of participants. A related study evaluated the effect of altruism in a medical context [29]. Subjects in three studies were interviewed about their reasons for participating in a study. There was no personal gain to participants in two of the three studies. The researchers concluded that the subjects' participation was mainly for the greater good. However, in each of these three studies, the participation may have been confounded by a personal look good feeling. There was no conflict in these studies between altruistic and look good feelings and so the differences between these two could not be measured. The authors also acknowledge this potential influence and refer to it as the potential to receive 'a warm glow' from participating. They refer to related work that looks at this type of altruism from an economic perspective via the donation of funds [30] instead of research participation.

A second subject-related bias is the *selection bias* or the *volunteer effect*. This bias may be encountered when the participants are volunteers [31] because there may be traits common in volunteers that are different from people who do not volunteer. Naturally, this may influence the findings. For example, the healthy volunteer bias [1] refers to overrepresentation of healthier participants in a study. This bias is especially pronounced in longitudinal studies. In addition to health, other personal characteristics may be overly present in a group of volunteers. In a formal study of selection bias, Adamis et al. [32] found that the method of getting elderly patients' informed consent for a mental health study had an enormous influence on the size and characteristics of the sample of participants. A formal capacity evaluation procedure followed by informed consent was compared to an informal procedure, which was "the usual" procedure, where informed consent and evaluating capacity were mingled. The formal procedure led to a smaller group of participants with less severe symptoms who agreed to participate and who were considered capable of making that decision.

Finally, a third well recognized subject-related bias is the *authorization bias*. This is the bias found when people need to authorize the use of their data for an observational study that does not require active participation in the study. Variations have been found when the informed consent process included a request for people to agree having their data included in a study. Kho et al. [33] found that differences existed between groups who consented and those who did not, but there was no systematic bias across all studies reviewed.

In addition to these known biases, there are other study participant characteristics that may form a bias and influence the study. Although these are more difficult to control, measuring the relevant characteristics may be helpful to identify outliers. For example, language skills are important. It is vital that participants understand the questions asked in a question-answer task or the items presented in a survey. Physical characteristics also should be considered. Participants may have difficulty using a mouse or clicking on scroll bars due to poor eyesight or tremors. Religion and political belief also may influence attitudes during testing. Measuring the study participants' relevant characteristics may serve as a pre-selection tool and help exclude non-representative people from participating. For example, in a study to measure the impact of various writing styles on understanding of health educational pamphlets, Leroy et al. [34, 35] excluded people with any medical background. Because the information presented was at the layman's level, any medical knowledge would have influenced the study's measurements of understanding. Other examples are required physical abilities to conduct the study as intended. For example, when designing visualization tools using 3D displays or colors in visualization, it is necessary to test the ability of participants to perceive 3D displays or see different colors.

Experimenter-Related Bias

Experimenter-related bias or *experimenter effects* are a type of bias related to experimenter behaviors that influence the outcomes or data. In most cases these effects are unintentional, and good experimental design or use of information technology can control many. There are two types of experimenter effects [24]: non-interactional and interactional experimenter effects. *Interactional experimenter effects* are those that lead to different behaviors or responses in the study participants due to the experimenter during the course of the study. The *non-interaction effects* are related to actions by the experimenter after the interaction with participants has been concluded.

Many interaction effects are not the results of dishonesty but of subtle cues that are given by the experimenter and picked up by the study participants. For example, an extra nod or more in-depth questions given during interviews may lead to better, longer or higher quality responses. An early and famous example is the Clever Hans effect. This effect is based on Clever Hans, a horse that could count. Oskar Pfungst determined that cues from his owner, who wasn't even aware of giving such cues, were responsible for the horse's abilities [36–38]. In the case of the horse, behaviors such as leaning forward when the count wasn't done yet and leaning backward when it was done helped the horse count. Current examples can be found in the many home videos of 'smart' pets. Another interactional experimenter effect is caused by personal characteristics of the facilitator that influence the participants. Gender, personal interaction styles, race, language skills and even personal hygiene are some of the many characteristics that may affect the outcome. Along the same lines, the topics or tasks covered may have an effect. People may be sensitive and prefer to avoid specific topics or may already be more or less biased before the experiment.

In addition to the biases that influence the interaction with participants, there exist *observer effects* or *non-interactional experimenter effects* that are the result of experimenter actions once the study has been executed. For example, different evaluation outcomes by different observers or evaluators demonstrate this effect. One evaluator may apply more lenient coding for the output of a new system. In most cases, this is unintentional.

Design-Related Bias

Some biases are inherent to the particular design used and cannot be attributed to subject or experimenter characteristics. One such design-related bias is the *placebo effect*, which is well known in medicine. It is an effect that can be attributed to participants believing that they are getting the treatment, even if they are not in reality getting any treatment.

In medicine, the placebo effect is significant when considering the importance of belief and mind over matter. Placebos are often used as the control condition in double-blind studies. Participants are given an inert pill, injection or treatment that looks the same as the experimental treatment. In some cases, the control condition has been found to have a positive effect even though no real treatment was provided. This placebo effect is therefore understood to be the effect of a control condition that is meant to be a placebo, without effect, but which has an effect after all. However, a note of caution is needed. The placebo effect found in medical studies may sometimes be more than a response bias and may be based on actual change in the brain or body [39].

In informatics, the use of a placebo control condition is difficult to accomplish. When evaluating an information system, it is not easy to organize a placebo condition where all interactions with a system are the same except for some interactions provided by the new system. Therefore, in informatics a different control condition is generally used: a baseline to compare the next system against. Since the baseline is usually the existing situation and often includes an existing system, it is incorrect to speak of a placebo effect.

A second design-related bias is a *carryover effect* or *contamination effect* which can be found when there are effects from the control condition that carry over to the experimental condition. It shows clearly how no experimental design is completely free of bias and the importance of choosing the best design for each study. The carryover effect is often a worry with within-subjects designs where study participants participate in multiple experimental conditions. For example, consider a validation study for a survey where each participant fills out two versions: the existing paper version and the new computerized version. The results of both versions are compared. With a within-subjects design, participants first start with one version of the survey and then complete the second version. However, it is very possible that experience with the first version influences the results of the second. For example, participants may try to repeat the same answers without really reflecting on the survey questions. This bias can be countered by counterbalancing the orderings, which is discussed in Chaps. 5 and 6.

A third design-related bias is the *second look bias*. This term, used in particular in medicine, refers to an effect similar to a carryover effect. It is encountered when study participants view data or an information system more than once and each time under different experimental conditions [34]. This bias especially needs to be taken into account with studies adopting a within-subjects design. Participants have an initial interaction with the system and learn about using the system or form an opinion about it. This first interaction will influence the second interaction. When they have a second look at the system, they may already have a better idea of how to use it efficiently, they may be less inclined to search for functions and so be more efficient (or give up faster on a task) or they may believe the system to be useless. This bias also can originate when the same data is reused over different experimental conditions.

Hawthorne Effect

The Hawthorne effect is one of the most famous biases and its discovery resulted in a set of books, commentaries, articles and many criticisms. In short and in its most simple terms, the Hawthorne effect is a change in behaviors that is supposed to be due to the knowledge that one is being measured or monitored.

The origin of this well known effect lies in a series of studies, conducted over several year, 1927–1932, at the Hawthorne Works of the Western Electric Company in Chicago [40, 41]. The studies started with five participants in the first few months, but soon many more workers, as many as 20,000 in total, participated and were interviewed. The experiments focused on worker conditions and efficiency by looking at changes such as rest pauses, shorter working days and wage incentives, among many other conditions. A general conclusion was that the changes in productivity were more due to the extra attention received and the knowledge that productivity was measured. However, these experiments were conducted in very different conditions from today: the tasks were monotone, the participants were females and many workers in those days had low levels of education. As such, there has been much debate over the years and caution is needed when generalizing these results [42]. It is doubtful the explanation is always as simple as a *measurement* or *attention effect*. Gale [43] shows how the context can help explain these effects.

The emerging use of informatics and technology in the realm of persuasion makes this effect a current topic again. It is said that 100% compliance, for example, with hand washing, can be accomplished with the placement of just one camera. Regardless of how simple or complex the effect may be, the term Hawthorne effect has stuck and is found frequently in educational and healthcare settings. For example, Leonard and Masatu [44] evaluate the impact of the presence of a research team on quality of care in Tanzania. They conclude that a Hawthorne effect is present with an increase of quality at the beginning of the team's presence, which over time gradually levels off to the same original levels. Conducting a randomized trial is no guarantee against a Hawthorne effect. Cook et al. [45] used self-reporting to measure the effects of an online versus print based diet and nutrition education program. They found significant improvements in both groups, regardless of the experimental conditions, and suggest this may be due to a Hawthorne effect.

Other Sources of Bias

There are other sources of variance and bias that cannot easily be categorized. One such source of variance that may result in bias is the availability of *identity information*. When doing studies, the identifying patient information is usually not present for privacy reasons. However, the identity of the treating physician may have an impact, especially when using historic cases. For example, when study participants consist of medical personnel, they may be acquainted with the treating physicians of the cases used in the study and they may put more or less trust in their own decisions for the case when seeing the decision by the known treating physician. This will influence how they work with each case and their willingness to make different decisions than the ones described in the case. Similarly, the study participants may have knowledge of the typical patients the treating physician works with and this may change their assumptions about the case and options for treatment.

The study environment factors are the characteristics of the environment that may affect the outcome of a study: characteristics associated with the room where the study is conducted, including noises, smells and temperature. Conducting experiments in a noisy room may prevent participants from concentrating and will affect many types of outcomes. Smelling the kitchen from a local restaurant may lead to participants hurrying through a self-paced study if they were hungry. An experimenter's personal characteristics or habits may affect the study. Some people are not aware of a personal smell and participants may feel uncomfortable when in close proximity during the study. Others may click their pen continuously during a study, annoying the participants. These environmental factors may introduce additional variance and affect the potential to see an effect of the experimental treatment. For example, when evaluating a visualization algorithm of health text [46], the author found that results from a first pilot study did not look promising. When scrutinizing the comments made by participants in response to an open question requesting comments on the algorithm, one of the subjects remarked that there was too much noise in the room when conducting the study. This led to a close look at the data for each experimenter which revealed that weaker results were attained by one of the two experimenters. It was discovered that after explaining the purpose of the study, this experimenter would spend the duration of the study time chatting with friends.

The unwanted effects resulting from bias can have serious consequences. Biases of a similar nature across all conditions may prevent the study from showing any results. Such studies may lead to a halt in follow-up research because no effect was found. When the bias arises in one but not other conditions, the consequences may be more serious and erroneous conclusions may be reached. Different systems or algorithms may be developed based on results from such studies.

References

1. Starks H, Diehr P, Curtis JR (2009) The challenge of selection bias and confounding in palliative care research. J Palliat Med 12(2):181–187
2. Kirk RE (1995) Experimental design: procedures for the behavioral sciences, 3rd edn. Brooks/Cole Publishing Company, Monterey
3. Rosson MB, Carroll JM (2002) Usability engineering: scenario-based development of human-computer interaction. interactive technologies. Morgan Kaufman Publishers, San Francisco
4. Gorini A, Pallavicini F, Algeri D, Repetto C, Gaggioli A, Riva G (2010) Virtual reality in the treatment of generalized anxiety disorders. Stud Health Technol Inform 154:39–43
5. Sidani S, Miranda J, Epstein D, Fox M (2009) Influence of treatment preferences on validity: a review. Can J Nurs Res 41(4):52–67
6. Friedman CP, Wyatt JC (2000) Evaluation methods in medical informatics. Springer-Verlag, New York
7. Maisiak RS, Berner ES (2000) Comparison of measures to assess change in diagnostic performance due to a decision support system. In: AMIA Fall Symposium, AMIA, pp 532–536
8. Goodman CS, Ahn R (1999) Methodological approaches of health technology assessment. Int J Med Inform 56:97–105
9. Kushniruk AW, Patel VL (2004) Cognitive and usability engineering methods for the evaluation of clinical information systems. J Biomed Inform 37:56–76
10. Brender J (2006) Handbook of evaluation methods for health informatics (trans: Carlander L). Elsevier Inc, San Diego
11. Kirakowski J (2005) Summative usability testing: measurement and sample size. In: Bias RG, Mayhew DJ (eds) Cost-justifying usability: an update for the Internet Age. Elsevier, Ireland, pp 519–553

12. Yousefi-Nooraie R, Irani S, Mortaz-Hedjri S, Shakiba B (2010) Comparison of the efficacy of three PubMed search filters in finding randomized controlled trials to answer clinical questions. J Eval Clin Pract [Epub ahead of print]. doi:10.1111/j.1365-2753.2010.01554.x

13. Kullo IF, Fan J, Jyotishman Pathak, Savova GK, Zeenat Ali, Chute CG (2010) Leveraging informatics for genetic studies: use of the electronic medical record to enable a genome-wide association study of peripheral arterial disease. J Am Med Inform Assoc 17(5):568–574

14. Wang B, Chen P, Zhang J, Zhao G, Zhang X (2010) Inferring protein-protein interactions using a hybrid genetic algorithm/support vector machine method. Protein Pept Lett 7(9):1079–84

15. Apostolopoulou E, Raftopoulos V, Terzis K, Elefsiniotis I.(2010). Infection probability score, APACHE II and KARNOFSKY scoring systems as predictors of bloodstream infection onset in hematology-oncology patients. BMC infectious diseases, 26(10):135

16. Hanauer DA, Miela G, Chinnaiyan AM, Chang AE, Blayney D (2007) The registry case finding engine: an automated tool to identify cancer cases from unstructured, free-text pathology reports and clinical notes. J Am Coll Surg 205(5):690–697

17. Witten IH, Frank E (2000) Data mining: practical machine learning tools and techniques with Java. The Morgan Kaufmann Series in data management systems. Morgan Kaufmann, San Francisco

18. Kirakowski J (1996) The software usability measurement inventory: background and usage. In: Jordan P, Thomas B, Weerdmeester B (eds) Usability evaluation in industry. Taylor and Francis, UK

19. Lewis JR (1995) IBM computer usability satisfaction questionnaires: psychometric evaluation and instructions for use. Int J Hum Comput Interact 7(1):57–78

20. Miller T (2008) Dynamic generation of a health topics overview from consumer health information documents and its effect on user understanding, memory, and recall. Doctoral Dissertation, Claremont Graduate University, Claremont

21. Leroy G, Chen H Med Textus (2002) An ontology-enhanced medical portal. In: Workshop on information technology and systems (WITS), Barcelona

22. Nance DW, Naps TL (1995) Introduction to computer science: programming, problem solving, and data structures, 3rd edn. West Publishing Company, Minneapolis/St. Paul

23. Xiao S, Bresler Y, Munson DC, Jr (2003). Fast Feldkamp algorithm for cone-beam computer tomography. In: 2003 international conference on image processing, IEEE, 14–17 September 2003, vol 813,pp II - 819–822, doi:10.1109/ICIP.2003.1246806

24. Rosenthal R, Rosnow RL (1991) Essentials of behavioral research: methods and data analysis. McGraw-Hill, Boston

25. Mast MS, Hall JA, Roter Dl (2007) Disentangling physician sex and physician communication style: their effects on patient satisfaction in a virtual medical visit. Patient Educ Couns 68:16–22

26. Sigall H, Aronson E, Hoose TV (1970) The cooperative subject: myth or reality? J Exp Soc Psychol 6(1):1–10. doi:doi:10.1016/0022-1031(70)90072-7

27. Adair JG, Schachter BS (1972) To cooperate or to look good?: the subjects' and experimenters' perceptions of each others' intentions. J Exp Soc Psychol 8:74–85

28. Rosnow RL, Suls JM, Goodstadt BE, Gitter AG (1973) More on the social pscyhology of the experiment: when compliance turns to self-defense. J Pers Soc Psychol 27(3):337–343

29. Dixon-Woods M, Tarranta C (2009) Why do people cooperate with medical research? findings from three studies. Soc Sci Med 68(12):2215–2222. doi:doi:10.1016/j.socscimed.2009.03.034

30. Andreoni J (1990) Impure altruism and donations to public goods: a theory of warm-glow giving. Econ J 100:464–477

31. Ammenwertha E, Gräber S, Herrmann G, Bürkle T, König J (2003) Evaluation of health information systems—problems and challenges. Int J Med Inform 71:125–135

32. Adamis D, Martin FC, Treloar A, Macdonald AJD (2005) Capacity, consent, and selection bias in a study of delirium. J Med Ethics 31(3):137–143

33. Kho ME, Duffett M, Willison D, Cook DJ, Brouwers MC (2009) Written informed consent and selection bias in observational studies using medical records: systematic review. BMJ 338:b866. doi:10.1136/bmj.b866

34. Leroy G, Helmreich S, Cowie J (2010) The influence of text characteristics on perceived and actual difficulty of health information. Int J Med Inform 79(6):438–449

35. Leroy G, Helmreich S, Cowie JR (2010) The effects of linguistic features and evaluation perspective on perceived difficulty of medical text. In: Hawaii international conference on system sciences (HICSS), Kauai, 5–8 January 2010

36. Baskerville JR (2010) Short report: what can educators learn from Clever Hans the Math Horse? Emerg Med Australas 22:330–331

37. Rosenthal R (1965) Clever Hans: the horse of Mr. von Osten. Holt Rinehart and Winston, Inc, Newyork

38. Pfungst O (1911) Clever Hans (The Horse of Mr. von Osten): a contribution to experimental animal and human psychology. Henry Holt and Company, New York

39. Price DD, Finniss DG, Benedetti F (2008) A comprehensive review of the placebo effect: recent advances and current thought. Annu Rev Psychol 59:565–590

40. Roethlisberger FJ, Dickson WJ (1946) Management and the worker, 7th edn. Harvard University Press, Cambridge

41. Landsberger HA (1958) Hawthorne revisited. Management and the worker, its critics, and developments in human relations in industry, vol IX. Corness studies in industrial and labor relations. W.F. Humphrey Press Inc, Geneva

42. Merrett F (2006) Reflections on the Hawthorne effect. Educ Psychol 26(1):143–146

43. Gale EAM (2004) The Hawthorne studies – a fable for our times? QJM Int J Med 97(7):439–449

44. Leonard K, Masatu MC (2006) Outpatient process quality evaluation and the Hawthorne effect. Soc Sci Med 63:2330–2340

45. Cook RF, Billings DW, Hersch RK, Back AS, Hendrickson A (2007) A field test of a web-based workplace health promotion program to improve dietary practices, reduce stress, and increase physical activity: randomized controlled trial. J Med Internet Res 9(2):e17. doi:doi:10.2196/jmir.9.2.e17

46. Miller T, Leroy G, Wood E (2006) Dynamic generation of a table of contents with consumer-friendly labels. In: American Medical Informatics Association (AMIA) Annual Symposium, Washington DC, 11–15 November 2006

Design Equation and Statistics

3

Chapter Summary

The previous chapter discussed the different types of variables one has to understand to design a study. This chapter uses the experimental design equation to show how these variables contribute to variability in results. The independent variable is assumed to affect the scores of the dependent variable. Other variables need to be controlled so that the effect of the independent variable can be clearly seen. Then, an overview of how to test the changes that the different levels of independent variables bring about is provided. Descriptive statistics are introduced first. These statistics describe the results, such as mean and standard deviation. Then inferential statistics or statistical testing follows. Statistical testing allows the researchers to draw conclusions about a population of users based on a study that involves a sample. Underlying, essential principles, such as the standard distribution and the central limit theorem, are reviewed, followed by the three tests most commonly performed in informatics: t-test, ANOVA and chi-square.

The effects of design choices on the study are also discussed. This includes a review of internal and external validity, errors and power. Internal validity refers to the degree to which a causal relation between the independent and dependent variables can be accepted. As such, the internal validity of a study relies on how well designed the study is. External validity refers to how well the conclusions of a study carry over to the environment where the system will be used. There are several threats to validity and alternative research designs to counter them. There is often a trade-off between internal and external validity. Studies that are more strongly controlled are usually less representative of "real life." Studies that are set up to resemble the actual environment more often suffer from less control.

The chapter concludes with a review of errors that can be made. Type I and Type II errors are explained together with the potential impacts of making such errors on research and development in different phases of system development. This section ends with a review of the power of studies to detect effects and the components in the study design that can be improved to increase the statistical power.

G. Leroy, *Designing User Studies in Informatics*, Health Informatics, DOI 10.1007/978-0-85729-622-1_3, © Springer-Verlag London Limited 2011

Experimental Design Model

Rationale

In informatics, the goal is to improve or change an existing condition by improving or adding an information system. When designing a study to evaluate whether this goal has been accomplished, hypotheses are stated that specify the relationship between the information system and the outcome. The hypotheses are about a population and specify which factors are expected to affect the outcome. If the hypotheses covered only one person or one group of persons, no statistical evaluation would be necessary. For example, if a researcher wanted to measure whether John lost weight by using a new weight loss support system, he could simply measure John's weight after a period and decide whether he lost weight or not. But most likely, the goal was to develop this new system for all people who need to lose weight, not for just one person.

To test hypotheses and draw conclusions about populations, an experiment is conducted with a sample of people. The sample is a subgroup of the population of interest. The population can be many different groups, for example, obese people, people with depression, children with autism, nurses in the emergency room and biomedical researchers. In informatics, the sample can also be a set of artifacts, for example, online community sites, personal health records and database queries. The observations made on the sample are used to approximate the population of interest. This is necessary because it is impossible to evaluate the system with all instances in a population. For example, it is practically impossible to test a weight loss support system with all people who need to lose weight.

Once the study has been conducted, the researcher collects the observations, or scores, for all participants in the different experimental conditions. These scores are combined; usually the average is taken for each experimental condition. However, there will be differences in the scores for individuals, even if they participated in the same experimental condition. The average score for a condition can therefore be seen as being comprised of different parts: a part of the score is due to the characteristics of the particular individual; a part is due to the experimental manipulation; and then a part is due to errors, random effects or unknown factors. The goal of a well designed study is to minimize the variations in scores due to errors or random effects and to maximize the variations due to the experimental condition.

The experimental design model ties all components together, using an equation to describe the factors that are expected to influence the outcome. The statistical tests are used to discover which of those components truly contributed to the outcome. The more appropriate the experiment design, the better the measurement of the treatment will be and the more valuable the conclusions about that treatment. This is because the observed score will include little variance due to errors and will mostly reflect the influence of the treatment.

Design Equation

The experimental design can be modeled using an equation. The notations used in this book are used in the behavioral sciences and adopted from Kirk [1]. For details on how to estimate each model parameter based on the sample observations, see Kirk [1]. The equation used in this chapter represents the simplest experimental design covered in this book: a completely randomized design. It is used to explain the principles. The equation later is adjusted for each different experimental design to show how experimental, nuisance and error effects can be distinguished from each other and estimated.

The design equation shows how an observed score gained during an experiment can be divided up into different parts. Each part represents a different fraction of the observed scores. It shows what affects an observation in an experiment and how systematic effects can be teased out. The independent, dependent and nuisance variables described in the previous chapter (Chap. 2) all have their place in this experimental design model.

The goal of an experiment is to find differences in scores for a dependent variable that are caused by exposure to the different levels of the independent variable. In this design equation, Greek symbols (α, μ, ε) are used to represent the population metrics, while the Latin alphabet (Y) is used to represent experimental observations. The components μ, α and ε represent the characteristics of the population. However, since it is impossible to measure every member of a population, these are estimated based on the sampled data.

The following equation (see Eq. 3.1) shows the components that make up the score of an individual in an experiment with one independent variable:

$$Y_{ij} = \mu + \alpha_j + \varepsilon_{i(j)} \tag{3.1}$$

1. The score Y represents the observed score that a participant achieved in one condition of the experiment. This formula shows that the score Y_{ij} is the observed score for individual i in condition j. It has three components.
2. μ (mu) is the overall mean. It is the score everyone in the population has in common, the average value around which the treatments vary.
3. α (alpha) represents the influence or the effect of the independent variable and is constant for all participants in one condition. It provides an adjustment of the overall mean due to the treatment j of the independent variable. The index j indicates which treatment or level of the independent variable this observation belongs to.
4. $\varepsilon_{i(j)}$ (epsilon) is the error term and it represents a further adjustment of the overall mean due to unwanted influences. These are the individual fluctuations that will be observed with each observation. The $\varepsilon_{i(j)}$ variation is due to unknown factors for individual i in condition j. The notation $i(j)$ is used to indicate that this change is specific to individual i in condition j (referred to as: i is nested within treatment j). If individual i participated in multiple conditions, this component would differ for that individual in the different conditions.

Table 3.1 Example of observed scores for weight loss program

	System 1	System 2
	Visualization approach	Text approach
	Y_{11} = kilograms lost by individual 1	Y_{12} = kilograms lost by individual 1
	Y_{21} = kilograms lost by individual 2	Y_{22} = kilograms lost by individual 2
	...	...
	Y_{n1} = kilograms lost by individual n	Y_{n2} = kilograms lost by individual n
Average	$\overline{Y}_1$ = average kilograms lost	$\overline{Y}_2$ = average kilograms lost

The following example is worked out to demonstrate this equation. Assume a weight loss program and the goal of the researchers is to find the best method to help obese patients lose weight. The independent variable is the encouragement approach used and it has two conditions: (1) a new, persuasive information system that uses visualization to display food intake and energy consumption and (2) an older information system that shows a textual summary of food intake and consumption. Since the goal is to lose weight, the dependent variable will be the weight loss in kilograms. Each person is measured at the beginning of the program and again after using the information system for 3 months. The metric of interest is the number of kilograms lost. Table 3.1 shows an overview of the observed scores.

The average score in each condition is the average of the individual scores. The mean in each condition is estimated by $\overline{Y}_j$ and calculated as shown in Eq. 3.2.

$$\overline{Y}_{.j} = \sum_{i=1}^{n} \frac{Y_{ij}}{n} \tag{3.2}$$

By applying the design equation to this example, it can be shown how each average score is composed of the following components:

μ or the population mean. This does not change between experimental conditions. For our example, assume that everyone would keep the same weight (no weight loss) and so μ would be zero for both experimental conditions. Each individual's weight loss is expected to vary around this mean.

α or the effect due to the experimental treatment. This component represents the influence of the experiment manipulation. Since α represents the independent variable, there are two possible values for j in this example: the new visualization system and the old text system. This is the main component of interest. The researchers want to see differences in this component for the two experimental conditions. For example, if one participant lost 5 kg with the new visualization system, this person's α would be 5. If all participants in the visualization condition lost a lot of weight, then the average score for this component would be high, for example, 5.5 kg weight loss: on average people lost weight in this condition. If participants in the text condition lost on average less weight, the α would be smaller, for example, 1.5 kg weight loss.

ε represents the error in the measurement. This is the third component, the error term that contributes to an individual's score. These variations can be due to numerous factors. One individual may have added weight because he had many parties to attend during the time of the experiment. Another individual started smoking and could control her eating habits better, so she lost more weight. Both are changes in weight not related to the experimental condition. It also is possible that different or incorrect scales were used to weigh people, resulting in additional small errors that are different for each person. Some people may have been measured after their meal while others may have been measured before their meal. If there are many changes in the score that are not due to the experimental condition, the error term will be large and it will be difficult to tease out the change in the observed weight due to the experimental condition. However, with good control of nuisance variables, by avoiding bias and with careful design, the error term can be made as small as possible.

To improve the user study design, the researcher needs to try to decrease the portion of the observed score that varies due to the error term and increase the portion that varies due to the experimental condition. For example, if some participants attend many parties and eat a lot, there will be considerable differences between participants. Those differences will not be due to the weight loss system but to the parties and the food served at those parties. Limiting the parties, for example, to one per week, would make the differences in error terms between individuals smaller. When the error is smaller, the contribution of the treatment to the observed scores will be larger. If there is a difference between experimental conditions, this will be more likely to emerge from the statistical analysis. The effects of smoking could also be controlled. For example, including only participants who do not smoke would help decrease the variance due to error. When the researcher is able to control such nuisance variables, the error term becomes smaller. If the proportion of a score due to the error term is smaller, it will be easier to see a significant effect of the experimental treatment.

Statistical Testing

Statistical testing is necessary to draw conclusions about a population with regard to the outcome of a treatment. Depending on how much is known about the population, how many conditions are being tested and the subject of the hypothesis (a difference between means or between variances) different statistics can be applied. The following section provides a brief overview of the rationale of statistical testing. This is followed by an introduction to important concepts including sample and population statistics, the central limit theorem and test statistics. This will suffice to understand and execute the procedures of a statistical evaluation. However, for a detailed description of these topics, the reader is referred to handbooks on statistics such as [2–9].

Descriptive and Inferential Statistics

When developing an information system, several persons will be observed who are using the new information system or who participate in a control condition. For each person and for each task that is performed, the researcher measures the outcome variables. Following this data collection, two sets of statistics are calculated: descriptive and inferential statistics.

Descriptive statistics are used to describe the values that were recorded for the study. A score is recorded for each individual and each task. Descriptive statistics are the metrics that provide an overview of the scores in the different experimental conditions. For example, the mean, maximum, minimum, standard deviation and median scores are descriptive statistics. *Inferential statistics*, in contrast, are used to reason from the specific to the general. These statistics need to be calculated to allow a researcher to make inferences about a population based on a sample of that population. Although variance is also a descriptive statistic, it is usually used to conduct an analysis of variance, not to simply describe the results.

When using statistical software, the researcher will find most of these descriptive statistics readily at her disposal. The two descriptive statistics most commonly used in reporting datasets are the mean and standard deviation. This pair provides a useful and effective description of a dataset. The *mean* is a descriptive statistic that measures central tendency. It is the arithmetic average of a set of N values (see Eq. 3.3) and shows the value around which all other values are centered. A "bar" on top of the symbol indicates this is a mean, for example, $\bar{x}$ is the mean of x.

$$\bar{x} = \frac{\sum_i^n x_i}{N} \tag{3.3}$$

The *standard deviation* (SD or σ) is another descriptive statistic; however, it is a measure of variability (see Eq. 3.4). It shows the dispersion of the values in the dataset.

$$SD = \sqrt{\frac{\sum_i^n (x_i - \bar{x})^2}{N}} \tag{3.4}$$

Essential Concepts

Below, an overview of essential concepts and their particular meaning in experimental design is provided. Understanding these concepts is necessary to comprehend statistical inference. Understanding statistical inference will help the researcher choose the best hypotheses and statistical tests and will improve the experimental design. The following concepts are briefly reviewed:
- Population, sample
- Test statistics, sample statistics, z-score

- Frequency distribution, normal distribution, standard normal distribution
- Central limit theorem
- Parametric and non-parametric tests
- Degrees of freedom.

The term *population* stands for an entire group of units that have characteristics in common. The goal of a study is to draw conclusions or make a statement about the population. In informatics this population can consist of people, events or artifacts, for example, the population of all children with autism, the population of all nurse practitioners or the population consisting of all PubMed abstracts. Parameters are used to describe the characteristics of a population. These are determined by measuring a sample of the population. The quality of a user study therefore often depends on the quality of the sample. Larger samples that are more representative are better. There are many different methods to acquire a sample to represent a population, for example random sampling or snowball sampling.

A *sample* is a subset of units measured. In statistical testing, the sample is intended to represent the entire population. In informatics, the sample can consist of people or it can consist of artifacts produced by people. For example, when testing a reminder system for diabetics, the intended population may be all diabetics. The sample will be a group of representative diabetics who participate in the study to test the system. In another example, researchers may be interested in testing a new algorithm that can detect statements in online community posts that indicate the person is depressed. In this case, the sample will not consist of the people who participate in online communities. Instead, the sample will consist of a set of online statements made by people.

A *test statistic* is used to test hypotheses about population parameters. While a parameter is a characteristic of a population, the test statistic is an estimate of this parameter. The t-test is an example of a test statistic. The choice of the test statistic depends on the hypothesis that is to be tested and what is known about the population.

A *sample statistic* is used to describe a characteristic of a sample of the population. It is a characteristic of a subset of units, for example, an average score of 50 subjects or the average number of words in clinical notes. In addition to plainly describing the sample, the sample statistic also can be used to estimate the characteristics of the entire population. Naturally, the sample statistic will be a better estimator when it is based on a larger sample and when the sample itself is more representative of the underlying population.

A *z-score*, also called *standard score* or *z-value* (see Eq. 3.5), indicates how many standard deviations a score is removed from the mean score. The formula below uses the population symbols for the mean and standard deviation because, to calculate z-scores, it is assumed that the population parameters are known. The z-score is a normalized score. It is especially useful when comparing scores for individuals who belong to different populations. For example, assume one wants to compare students who have taken an entrance exam. If two students have taken the exam in different years, it is difficult to compare their scores. The difficulty of the exam may differ from year to year. As a result, the actual scores of the students

Fig. 3.1 Normal distribution

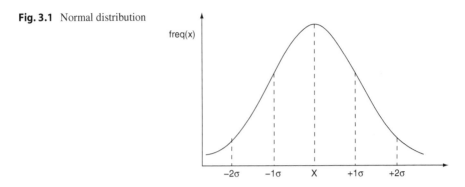

are not very useful in a comparison. A z-score, however, makes it possible to compare these values after all. The z-score compares the score against the average for the group, making comparisons over samples more meaningful. Note that the population consists of all students who took the exam in each year and so the population mean and standard deviation are known, as required for calculating z-scores. The z-score is calculated as follows:

$$z = \frac{(X - \mu)}{\sigma} \tag{3.5}$$

A *frequency distribution* shows how values are dispersed. It shows the scores, the x-values, on the x-axis and the frequency of occurrence of these values (*freq(x)*) on the y-axis. The *normal distribution* is the name for the distribution that is often referred to as the bell curve (see Fig. 3.1). The normal distribution is completely defined when the mean and the standard deviation are known. It is a frequency distribution with special characteristics: it is symmetrical, extends to infinity on both sides and the area under the curves adds up to 1. This area is used to estimate the probability of values, which can be done in terms of the standard deviation: 68% of the area will be between one standard deviation to the left and to the right of the mean and 95% of the area will be between two standard deviations to the left and to the right of the mean. This means that 95% of the values fall within two standard deviations of the mean. The *standard normal distribution* is a normal distribution with a mean of 0 and a standard deviation of 1. A normal distribution can be converted to a standard normal distribution by converting the scores to z-scores.

The *central limit theorem* describes how samples taken from a population are distributed. Assume there is a population of which the mean is μ and the standard deviation is σ. When a sample is taken from this population, the sample mean can be calculated. When such sampling is done many times, the frequency of the means can be drawn as a distribution. The central limit theorem states that when enough samples are drawn from a population, their means will be distributed as in a normal distribution. The larger the sample size, the better the distribution will approximate the normal distribution. It is essential to understand that it is the sample size that is important and not the number of samples. This normal distribution (with a sufficiently large sample size) is achieved even for non-normal, underlying distributions. If a distribution is skewed, the distribution of the means will still approach the normal distribution if the sample size is large enough. (Note: searching online for "central limit theorem simulation" will result in a list of simulations that show very clearly this relation between sample size and distribution.)

Parametric and nonparametric tests are both useful for statistical testing. The t-test and ANOVA are examples of parametric tests. They involve the estimation of population parameters and use the mean values of observations. They also require specific assumptions about the distributions to be met, such as normality. Nonparametric tests do not relate to population parameters and are used for data that is not at interval or ratio level but at nominal or ordinal level. Chi-square is an example of such a test. Although there are still requirements that need to be met, such as independent observations, this test relies on frequencies of observations in a sample, not a mean value.

Degrees of freedom (*df*) is used to define how many values in a sample can vary. For example, assume a sum of two values. If one value and the sum are known, then the second value cannot vary anymore, it is known. There is only one degree of freedom. Degrees of freedom are an important concept in test statistics such as the t-test.

Rationale of Statistical Testing

When conducting an experiment, a researcher intends to make a statement about a population. The goal is not limited to describing the sample of people and how they reacted to a treatment, but to make statements about how all people who belong to the population of interest would react to the treatment. Statements about the population need to be inferred from the data gained from the sample. For example, assume a decision support system that has been installed in a hospital to improve a physician's ability to correctly recognize brain tumors without invasive tests. The goal of a user study is not limited to finding whether more correct decisions were made by the physicians who participated in the study, but to generalize any findings to all physicians who would use the decision support system. Because of this wish to draw conclusions about the population of all physicians based on results achieved with only a sample of a few physicians, statistical inference is needed.

To conduct an experiment, hypotheses about the effect of a treatment on a population are detailed. These hypotheses show the relationship between the independent variable, the treatment, and the dependent variable, the outcome. For example, a research hypothesis for the decision support system to recognize brain tumors could be that less than 1% of brain tumors are missed as a result of using the system. Another example hypothesis would be that surgeons using the decision support system make more correct decisions than those who do not have the decision support system.

For each research hypothesis, two statistical hypotheses are stated: the null hypothesis and the alternative hypothesis. They are mutually exclusive. The null hypothesis states that there is no effect of the treatment. It is essential to state hypotheses in this manner because one cannot prove a hypothesis to be true. One can only prove it to be wrong. This is because it is impossible to test all data points that make up a population. Therefore, it is impossible to prove that something is true for all instances. However, it is possible to show that a hypothesis is false by showing at least one example where this falsity exists. So, if a condition shows that the null hypothesis is false, it needs to be rejected. Since the null hypothesis and the alternative hypothesis are mutually exclusive, rejecting the null hypothesis means accepting the alternative hypothesis. The alternative hypothesis states the effect: it can be concluded there was an effect of the independent variable on the dependent variable.

Statistics are used to decide whether the null hypothesis can be rejected or not. There are two types of hypotheses. In one type, the hypothesis is about a value: a treatment is compared against a number, for example, achieving fewer than five mistakes. In the other type, the hypothesis is about a comparison of conditions: treatments are compared against each other, for example, making a decision with the aid of a decision support system versus making the decision without that decision support system.

If the hypothesis is about a given value, the researcher obtains a random sample of units from the population and calculates the mean. This sample is intended to represent the population about which the conclusions will be made. For example, the sample could consist of 20 surgeons who evaluate medical records of patients with suspected brain tumors over a year. The decisions they make are tracked and compared against biopsy results. The mean for the dependent variable, e.g., the number of correct decisions, is calculated. The null hypothesis states that 1% or more of brain tumors are missed. For these values, the test statistic, such as the t-statistics, is calculated as shown in the next section. Then, the probability of finding that value for the test statistic is calculated. These probabilities are known and can be looked up in tables or are provided by the statistical software being used. The probability shows how rare it would be that the null hypothesis was true given that number. If the probability of finding this test statistic is very small, say smaller than 5%, the hypothesis is rejected. The probability for rejection is stated in advance and is referred to as the significance level or α. If the null hypothesis for the example is rejected, it can be concluded that errors made were less than 1%.

If the hypothesis is about two conditions, the same rationale is followed. Two samples are obtained, one for each condition. For example, the sample could consist of 20 surgeons who use the decision support system and 20 others who do not use the system. Their decisions are tracked and compared. The number of correct decisions of each group is recorded. A test statistic, for example the t-statistic, is calculated using those two means. Then, the probability of finding this statistic is looked up and if it is smaller than a predefined value, for example 5%, then the null hypothesis is rejected. This means that there is a small chance, 5% or less, that this value could be found while the null hypothesis is true. Since the chance is so small, the null hypothesis is rejected and the alternative hypothesis is accepted.

t-test

The t-test relies on Student's t-distribution, first described by W.S. Gosset. Gosset was a chemist working in a brewery who published his work under the alias "Student." The alias has remained and the distribution is referred to as Student's t-distribution. The t-test is a parametric test used with hypotheses about two means of populations. When more means need to be compared, it is necessary to conduct an Analysis of Variance (ANOVA). The t-test is used when the population standard deviation is not known and needs to be estimated from the sample.

Although the t-test is a straightforward test, its calculations are adjusted to take different experimental designs into account. The formulas are adjusted for different sampling methods, equal or unequal numbers of observations in each group, equal or unequal variances in each group and the assumed directionality of the effect. For the discussion below, we assume equal sample sizes and variances. Small variations in the formulas are needed when this is not the case. Statistical software will take care of these variations, as long as the user indicates them when running the software. The general case is described below.

When multiple samples are drawn from a population and t is calculated for each, the distribution of these values assumes a t-distribution. The t-distribution is referred to as a family of distributions because its shape changes. With increasing sample size (n), the t-distribution approximates the normal distribution. From this it follows that the area under the curve of the t-distribution approaches that of a normal distribution. As a result, the distribution can be used to estimate how rare a value is. As explained above, in statistical testing a hypothesis is rejected when the associated t-value is very rare.

Below, three approaches to calculate t are described. These are the most common designs used in informatics. The first approach is used when the study aims to test whether a sample mean differs from a hypothesized mean μ_0. The numerator describes the difference between the sample and the hypothesized population mean. The denominator describes the standard deviation or how much variation could be expected by chance. We assume here that the sample sizes are equal so that n, the sample size, is used to calculate the degrees of freedom. For this test, the t-statistic is calculated as is shown in Eq. 3.6:

$$t = \frac{\bar{x} - \mu_0}{\frac{S}{\sqrt{n}}} \tag{3.6}$$

The denominator of this formula is calculated as is shown in Eqs. 3.7 and 3.8:

$$S = \sqrt{\frac{\sum_{i=1}^{n}(x_i - \bar{x})^2}{df}} \tag{3.7}$$

$$df = n - 1 \tag{3.8}$$

The t-test can also be used to compare two sample means. In this case, there are two variants depending on the sampling method used to assign subjects to experimental conditions. When the subjects are assigned in random fashion to one of two conditions an *independent samples t-test* is conducted. With this t-test, it is assumed that there is no relationship between the items in the first sample and those in the second sample, for example, when study subjects will only participate in one experimental condition. This design is discussed in detail in Chap. 4. When comparing two conditions, t is calculated as described in Eq. 3.9. The numerator has been replaced by the subtraction, "the comparison," of the two means of interest, and the denominator has also been adjusted to take into account that there are two samples (see Eq. 3.10). Note that equal sample sizes are assumed: n is used in the denominator.

$$t = \frac{\overline{x}_1 - \overline{x}_2}{\frac{S_{x_1 x_2}}{\sqrt{n}}} \tag{3.9}$$

$$S_{x_1 x_2} = \sqrt{(S_{x_1})^2 + (S_{x_2})^2} \tag{3.10}$$

When there is a natural pairing, a relationship between the subjects in the two conditions, a *paired samples or dependent samples t-test* is appropriate. Such pairings can be of different types. For example, one such pairing could be based on a relationship between the subjects, such as when the effects of marriage therapy are evaluated on both husbands and wives. In one experimental group, the husbands are measured and in the other the wives. The husbands and wives are related and so a paired sample design will be appropriate. In other cases, the relationship does not result from a real-world association between subjects. Subjects in different experimental conditions can be paired based on characteristics they share that are relevant to the experiment. For example, in experiments to reduce the number of cigarettes smoked, a subject in the control condition who smokes 1 to 5 cigarettes per day could be paired with a similar subject in the experimental condition, while a subject who smokes 20–25 cigarettes per day in the control condition should be paired with a similar subject in the experimental condition.

The extreme version of this design with paired subjects is found when all subjects participating in the first experimental condition also participate in the second condition. This is called a *repeated measures* design because the measures are repeatedly taken from the same subjects. For example, evaluating the effectiveness of the decision support system to detect brain tumors could be conducted over a long period of time: for the control condition, the surgeons are first studied when making decisions without the decision support system; for the experimental condition, the same surgeons are studied when they make decisions with the decision support system. The same group of surgeons participates in both conditions. The first 6 months, the results without a decision support system are collected and the following 6 months,

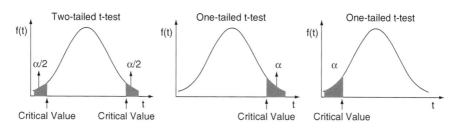

Fig. 3.2 Critical values for one- and two-tailed t-tests

the results with a decision support system are collected. This design is addressed in detail in Chap. 5 where within-subject designs are discussed.

For the paired samples t-test, t is calculated differently (see Eq. 3.11). The numerator and denominator are adjusted to represent the differences between the two measures for each sampling unit; t is now calculated based on the difference between two scores (see Eq. 3.12).

$$t = \frac{\bar{x}_D - \mu_D}{\dfrac{S_D}{\sqrt{n}}} \tag{3.11}$$

$$x_D = x_2 - x_1 \tag{3.12}$$

The following steps in the statistical evaluation are the same regardless of the type of t-test that was conducted. Once t has been calculated, it is compared against a critical value. This critical value represents the probability where it would become rare for the hypothesis to be true. If t is larger than this critical value, it would be very rare that the null hypothesis is true and so it can be rejected.

The critical values differ for one-tailed and two-tailed t-tests. A one-tailed t-test is appropriate when the hypothesis includes directionality, for example, when hypothesizing that using the decision support system will lead to more correct decisions by the surgeons. This is a directional prediction that is shown as a ">" or "<" in the hypotheses. A two-tailed t-test is appropriate when there is no directionality and the hypotheses are about equality, for example, when hypothesizing that the number of correct decisions made by surgeons will be different with the decision support system compared to without. It does not specify how the decision will differ: more or less correct.

Figure 3.2 shows how the directionality of the hypothesis affects the critical values against which the calculated t-value will be compared. With a two-tailed t-test, the critical values exist on either side of the mean and their combined value is equal to α or the probability at which an outcome is considered rare. With a one-tailed t-test, the critical value exists only on one side of the mean. In this case, the critical value that needs to be reached for the t-value to be considered rare will be lower. This will have an effect on the power of the study, which is explained in the last section of this chapter.

Naturally, there are assumptions made when using the t-test. The most important of these is that the data is normally distributed. Although no exact numbers can be given, it is fairly safe to assume that the normal distribution is achieved when the sample is large enough, which is usually the case when $n > 30$ [1]. According to some, the t-test is fairly robust against deviations from these assumptions. For example, with equal sample sizes, a moderate deviation from normality may still result in valid conclusions [10]. In the examples above, it was assumed that the variances and sample sizes are equal. However, when this is not the case, adjustments can be made in how t is calculated.

To maximize t and increase the chance that a significant effect is detected when it exists, there are three strategies that should be taken into account. Since these strategies are common to t-tests and ANOVA, in fact they are true for all experimental designs, a detailed discussion on how to accomplish this is provided in Chap. 14. Only a brief summary is provided here. The first important strategy is to increase the distance between the means of the different conditions. This can be done by choosing the best possible treatments to compare with the base level. When that distance is larger, the t-value also will be larger. The second important strategy is to decrease the variability within each treatment group. The variability between the groups then becomes easier to detect, and this will lead to more significant results. This can be accomplished by reducing the variability of characteristics that are associated with the dependent variable, in other words, by making the sample units homogeneous so they only differ with respect to their response to treatments. The third strategy is to increase the effect size of the study. This can be done by choosing treatments with large effects and by increasing the sample size.

F-test and ANOVA

The previous section described the t-test to compare two means. When there are only two means to be compared, the t-test and the F-test lead to the same conclusions about rejecting the null hypothesis; both tests are interchangeable. However, in many cases, there are more than two experimental conditions and so more than two means need to be compared. One could carry out a t-test for every possible combination, but this would increase the chances of making a Type I error and rejecting the null hypothesis incorrectly. Therefore, it is better to use the F-test as part of an Analysis of Variance (ANOVA). ANOVA can be seen as an extension of the t-test for more than two treatments. The F-test can be used to test hypotheses about variances of populations and to test hypotheses about the means of populations. The latter is the more common use of the test.

The F-measure uses the variance to evaluate hypotheses about means and is intuitively easy to understand. For example, when a new information system is compared with an old system, the variation between groups (those who use the old versus the new system) is expected to be higher than the variation within each group.

In other words, if a system has an effect, the difference between the group with and the group without the system would be larger than the differences in each group. The F-measure applies this insight and is calculated as the ratio of the variation between the groups to the variation within each group.

For example, assume an experiment with one independent variable, namely a computer based meditation program to help people sleep longer and better. The participants who are recruited are all volunteers who report that they usually sleep only 4–5 h without waking up. There are three experimental conditions: one-third of the participants use the program, one-third reads a book before going to bed and one-third does not receive special instructions. Participants are assigned to one of the three conditions by random selection. The number of hours slept is recorded for each participant. ANOVA is used to calculate whether there is more variation between the two groups than within each group. If this independent variable has an effect, it can be assumed that the difference in the number of hours slept will differ more between the three groups. If the researcher is lucky, the group using his meditation program will sleep much longer and better than the other two groups.

The *F-test* is a general test that compares multiple means with one general comparison. As such, it does not increase the chances of making a Type I error when comparing multiple conditions. When there is one independent variable, this test is called a *one-way ANOVA*. For example, assume that the sleep experiment includes four conditions: the meditation program, the book reading, an hour of yoga and a condition without any of these. These are the four experimental conditions across one independent variable: sleep intervention. The researcher conducts a one-way ANOVA to evaluate the effects on the number of hours slept. He hypothesizes that the means are equal for the different conditions; this is the null hypothesis. If the result of this ANOVA indicates a significant effect of the treatment, the researcher can reject the null hypothesis. However, the ANOVA results do not specify which means differ from each other. It is possible that all means differ from each other or it could be that only two means differ from each other. The researcher will need to conduct post hoc tests to pinpoint which means differ significantly.

An F-test will indicate a significant difference when there is more variation between the groups ($MS_{Between\ Groups}$, MS_{BG} or MSBG) than variation within in each group ($MS_{Within\ Groups}$, MS_{WG} or MSWG). Eq. 3.13 describes the relationship between the two: the numerator should be larger than the denominator when there is a significant effect of a treatment. MS stands for "mean square" and is used to estimate the population variance for a given population or experimental condition. The variance described by the numerator is the estimated variance due to the experimental effect and the error variance. The variance described by the denominator is the estimated variance due to the error variance only. The F-measure is calculated as follows:

$$F = \frac{MS_{BG}}{MS_{WG}} \tag{3.13}$$

The mean square values (MS) are calculated by dividing the sum of squares (SS) by the appropriate degrees of freedom (see Eq. 3.14).

$$MS = \frac{SS}{df} \tag{3.14}$$

The calculation of SS relies on the principle that the total sum of squares (Total SS) is made up of the sum of squares between (Between SS) and the sum of squares within conditions (Within SS) as is shown in Eq. 3.15. Equations 3.15–3.18 show how each term is calculated. The total variance (Eq. 3.16) describes the summed variation of each individual value compared to the means of the condition means ($\bar{M}$). The variance within a condition (Eq. 3.17) is the sum of squares within each condition comparing the individual scores to the condition mean. M_k represents the mean in the kth condition. The variance between conditions (Eq. 3.18) is the sum of squares between conditions comparing the mean of each condition to the total mean.

$$SS_{Total} = SS_{Between} + SS_{Within} \tag{3.15}$$

$$SS_{Total} = \sum_{i}^{N}(x_i - \bar{M})^2 \tag{3.16}$$

$$SS_{Within} = \sum_{i}^{k}(x_i - M_k)^2 \tag{3.17}$$

$$SS_{Between} = \sum_{i}^{k}(n_k(M_k - \bar{M})^2) \tag{3.18}$$

The F-statistic is used in the same manner as the t-statistic and is calculated for the observed values in the samples. There are critical values associated with reaching a specified significance level for a given number of degrees of freedom. When the F-value is larger than the critical value, the null hypothesis can be rejected.

There are assumptions underlying ANOVA that have to be met. These assumptions are often expressed in terms of the errors or the deviation of each score from the mean. First of all, the errors need to be independent from each other, in other words, the sample needs to be gained by random sampling. The errors also need to display homogeneity of variance, in other words, equal variances are assumed for the different conditions. And finally, the errors need to be normally distributed. According to Rosenthal and Rosnow [11], the most important condition to be met to allow valid conclusions is the random and independent sampling of units (independence of errors), but F is considered robust for violations against the other two assumptions. For a detailed discussion of the consequences of violating these assumptions, see Kirk [1].

Although there are many similarities between the t-test and the F-test, the F-test provides more options and can be adjusted to many more experimental study designs. Similar to the t-test, the F-test can be used for between- and within-subject designs. Depending on which design is chosen, the denominator of the F-test will be calculated differently. In addition, a fixed effects model or random effects model can be assumed, which will use different calculations of the error variances. With a fixed effects model, the treatments that are evaluated are assumed to be all the ones that are of interest to the researcher. Conclusions about rejecting the null hypothesis are limited to those treatments. With a random effects model, the treatments are assumed to be a random sample of all possible treatment levels that are of interest. The calculations of F differ for both models, and the researcher can typically choose which model to use within a statistical software package.

Finally, the F-distribution differs depending on the degrees of freedom. This is similar to the t-test but more complicated, since with the F-distribution two types of degrees of freedom affect the shape of the distribution: the numerator or between-groups and the denominator or within-groups degrees of freedom. These will affect the critical value for F that needs to be reached to reject the null hypothesis at a specified α. The reader is referred to statistical manuals [1, 3–5, 8, 9] for a detailed description and worked out examples of these calculations.

Chi-Square

The previous two sections described the t-test and the ANOVA, which compare the means of experimental conditions. Chi-square is a different type of test. It is a non-parametric test that is used to compare frequency counts of observations. These frequencies can be thought of as counts of characteristics of units, such as gender, or counts of categories, such as answers to multiple choice questions. It is important to understand the difference between frequencies and means. With chi-square, counts for the possible values of a variable are compared, not the scores themselves. It is used when there are two or more variables that are expected to influence each other. In other words, it tests whether the distribution of characteristics is random or influenced by the variables. When it is used with one variable, the test is also called the *chi-square test for goodness of fit* because it evaluates whether an observed distribution fits an expected distribution. When it is used to test whether there is a relationship between two or more variables, the test is also called the *chi-square test for independence*.

Chi-square can be used with one or more nominal or ordinal variables. Nominal variables are variables that have categories that are different but are not meant to be ordered. For example, gender has two possible labels (male and female) or possibly three labels: male, female, unknown. Other examples are occupation, treatment level, native language or race. However, there are many nominal variables that are commonly included in experiments. For example, choosing a preference with a multiple choice question is a good example of a nominal variable. Ordinal variables are variables where the categories can be ordered as higher or lower. For example, letter grades, A–F. Both nominal and ordinal variables are often included as part of surveys and so answers to multiple choice survey questions are suitable for this type of testing.

Table 3.2 Example contingency tables

A	Gender			B	Gender		
Smoking habits	Male	Female	Total	Smoking habits	Male	Female	Total
Smokers	35	35	70	Smokers	45	25	70
Non-smokers	15	15	30	Non-smokers	5	25	30
Total	50	50		Total	50	50	

Chi-square is most easily explained with a contingency table and an example. In Table 3.2, two variables are shown that represent the answer to two survey questions. The first variable is the gender of the respondents and has two categories: male and female. Assume that every respondent answered the gender question. The second variable is about the smoking habits of the participant. Assume that two choices were provided: smoker or non-smoker. A chi-square test can be conducted to test whether gender and smoking habits are related. It could be hypothesized that gender influences whether participants smoke or not. Naturally, the null hypothesis states that this is not the case and that the frequency of smoking or not is not influenced by gender.

Table 3.2 shows two possible outcomes of presenting the survey to 100 persons. Table 3.2A shows frequencies that indicate that there are more smokers than non-smokers (70% smokers), but the ratio of smokers to non-smokers is the same for both genders. In other words, the proportion of smokers versus non-smokers is not systematically influenced by gender and the null hypothesis cannot be rejected. Table 3.2B, in contrast, shows how the proportions could have been very different. In part B, there are many more males who are smokers; however, there are an equal number of smokers and non-smokers in the female group. In this case, the null hypothesis will be rejected. Gender has an effect on smoking habits.

Chi-square is used to test two types of null hypothesis. The first type, very commonly used, is found when the distribution is expected to be random or equal. This is also called the *no-preference null hypothesis* [3]. For example, we usually expect an equal number of men and women in a sample. When the null hypothesis is rejected, this means that the frequencies are not equal. The second type of null hypothesis is used when there are known distributions in a population. The expected frequencies should reflect this known distribution. For example, assume a distribution that specifies the ratio of American adults with a completed degree as follows (note: these numbers are roughly based on 2009 Census data for California), 10% have a graduate degree, 30% have an undergraduate degree and 60% do not have a 4 year degree. When a study is conducted, the educational degrees achieved by the study participants can be compared with these expected frequencies. The null hypothesis states that the education of the people in the sample will be distributed in the same manner as the population. However, if the sample differs from these expected frequencies, the null hypothesis will be rejected.

In medicine, chi-square is often used to demonstrate that a sample was appropriate for the study and that experimental controls were carried out successfully. The presence of people with certain characteristics in experimental conditions is compared among groups, not the scores of these people on some test. It is used to demonstrate the lack of a systematic relationship, in other words, random sampling succeeded and participants with different characteristics were equally present in the different experimental conditions. For example, Smith et al. [12] used it to evaluate whether the proportion of patients adhering to a treatment was the same in the treatment and the placebo group.

Chi-square (χ^2) is calculated by comparing observed frequencies of dependent measures with expected frequencies (see Eq. 3.19). For each cell of a contingency matrix, the difference is calculated between the expected frequency (E) of membership and the observed frequency (O) relative to that expected frequency. The differences are summed. As a result, chi-square describes the discrepancy between what is expected and what is observed.

$$\chi^2 = \sum_{i=1}^{k} \frac{(O_i - E_i)^2}{E_i} \tag{3.19}$$

The larger this number, the more like there is big discrepancy between what is expected and what is observed. How large such a value should be for the null hypothesis to be rejected depends on the χ^2 distribution being used. When there are more categories, the values will be larger and so the critical value should also be larger. Therefore, a different χ^2 distribution is used depending on the number of categories. More specifically, the distributions differ depending on the degrees of freedom. For example, when there are four categories for one variable, the degrees of freedom are three $(df=3)$; when there are two variables each with three categories, the degrees of freedom are four $(df=2 * 2=4)$. In general, the degrees of freedom for two variables in a contingency table are calculated as shown in Eq. 3.20:

$$df = (rows - 1) * (columns - 1) \tag{3.20}$$

Similar to the t-test and ANOVA discussed above, assumptions are made when doing a chi-square test. A first requirement for having a valid test is that the units need to have been independently and randomly selected. Furthermore, each unit can only appear in one cell of the contingency table. So, for the example with smokers and non-smokers, no participant can be included in the dataset who indicates both "smoker" and "non-smoker" as their answer. In practice, this needs to be taken into account when designing survey questions. Survey questions where participants can indicate more than one answer to a question ("check all that apply") cannot be analyzed using chi-square. One possible workaround is to dummy code that variable and have a separate category for all those who checked multiple answers. A further requirement for conducting chi-square analysis is that frequencies need to be sufficiently large. There are different guidelines on what constitutes sufficiently large frequencies. In general, it is advised that most cells should have an expected frequency of more than five and no cells should have an expected frequency of one or zero. However, according to others, reasonable results can be achieved with expected frequencies as small as one as long as the total number of observations is high enough [11].

Significance Levels

All tests above rely on critical values that need to be met for a significance level α to be reached. However, the increased use of statistical software is changing how α is reported. Originally, most journal and conference editors, and most professional societies, required the reporting of significance levels as either significant or not significant. Common cutoff levels used were a p-value of 0.05 or smaller values such as 0.01. However, exact p-values are becoming the norm. This is because these cutoff levels are artificial boundaries. In addition, it is now easy to calculate α using software packages. More exact p-values definitely impact the results interpretation. For example, achieving a p-value of 0.051 would be considered "not significant" with a 0.05 cutoff value. However, if this result was achieved with a relatively small sample, it would be a very useful indicator that a significant effect can be expected with a larger sample. In contrast, if a p-value of 0.9 was found, this is a clear indication that there was no effect. Simply reporting "significant" or "not significant" does not allow this type of interpretation.

Internal Validity

The focus of this section is on internal validity. There exist others types of validity that can be measured but they are not the focus of this book. For example, to measure psychological characteristics or traits of people, surveys are most often used and the validity measures of interest are construct validity (how well a survey measures that psychological characteristic), content validity and criterion validity (both concurrent and predictive).

Internal validity refers to the degree that statements about the independent variable causing the effects in the dependent variable can be accepted as valid or true. Threats to internal validity are bias and confounding. The goal of designing a true experiment with randomization of subjects to experimental conditions is to ensure, as much as possible, internal validity. However, since it is impossible to measure everything, absolute internal validity does not exist. Providing an exhaustive list of the threats to internal validity is not possible. But several threats are common to many studies and so being aware of them will help the researcher counter them or take them into account when forming conclusions from the experimental data.

Some common threats to internal validity in all types of studies are history and maturation. *History* as a threat to internal validity stands for the possibility that something happens between administration of the treatment and measurement of the dependent variable. When something happens in between those two events, the causal relationship between the two cannot be shown in many cases. *Maturation* refers to processes that appear due to time passing. Both can be controlled are taken into account with proper designs. For example, Heywood and Beale [13] worked with children diagnosed with attention deficit/hyperactivity disorder and trained them using biofeedback and a control condition to reduce behavioral symptomatology. They used a single-case design and alternated conditions between the treatment and control. By using the subjects as their own control and alternating treatments, using an AABAB pattern where A was the control and B the treatment condition, they could avoid the possibility that maturation or history affected participants in one condition.

Other threats to internal validity are more specific to medicine, for example, mortality and treatment preference. *Mortality* refers to the loss of subjects in an experimental condition that changes the distribution of subject characteristics in a condition. Mortality can especially be a problem with severely ill patients who become too sick to participate or pass away; or if there is turnover in clinical personnel when clinicians are the study participants. *Treatment preference* is a bias due to the belief that some treatments are more desirable and so are preferred to other treatments; usually the placebo conditions or older treatments are not desirable. Interestingly, treatment preference is a general characteristic of the population and its environment. It has therefore been argued that external validity suffers when this treatment preference is ignored [15]. According to others, there is no evidence for such a claim. For example, Leykin et al. [14] focused on this treatment preference with patients suffering from depression. Participants were asked if they preferred antidepressant medication or cognitive therapy as their treatment. Half of the participants where then randomly assigned to their preferred treatment and the other half their non-preferred treatment. The authors found no effect on the reduction of depressive symptoms as a result of this preference.

External Validity

External validity refers to the degree that the results of the study with its given sample can be generalized to the entire population. There are four aspects that need to be considered for their effects on external validity: the users, the environment, the data or information used and the system tested. The more the sample resembles the reality with regard to these aspects, the more external validity the study will have. Unfortunately, there is often a trade-off between internal and external validity. Making a situation more realistic or placing the study in its intended environment usually will come at the cost of some control. Negotiating this trade-off between internal and external validity is part of experimental design.

Users

The users who participate in the study should be representative of the intended users of the information system or algorithms. By working with representative users, the results will be representative of what can be expected in the field. For example, working with volunteers to evaluate a new information system may limit the generalizability because of a selection bias. Volunteers may be people who enjoy trying out new technology and so may be overly positive about any new technology. Representative users also will be more willing to participate in the study and give serious feedback. In contrast to volunteers, users who are not seriously interested in a system will not use and test the system seriously.

In medicine, it is common to have inclusion and exclusion criteria to define the user group. The larger this list, the more specific the user group becomes. When the selection criteria define a group very narrowly and strictly, the study results will be increasingly limited and not generalizable. However, in many cases, they may still have high validity for this group and may be very valuable. For example, when developing an information system for children with autism who are nonverbal, the results of the study will not apply to all children with autism. However, since there are many children who belong to this group, this study would still be very valuable.

In informatics, there are additional advantages to working with representative users. By working with users and conducting studies, developers have an opportunity to get feedback on the system that goes beyond a statistical evaluation and may help guide future developments or expansion of the software. Good software depends on more than only theories that can be studied. It also needs users who will use the system while being naïve about the underlying theories. Working with these users will lead to many valid and interesting comments and suggestions that will be very valuable to the development and marketing teams.

Environment

The environment is a very important factor and often difficult to mimic when an information system is studied in a laboratory. Even seemingly straightforward comparisons between systems, e.g., for image comparison, may suffer if not carried out in natural settings. For example, in real job situations, people may answer the phone or respond to email while evaluating images. Many parallel processes are going on that are not part of the laboratory study. The researcher should weigh the impact such environmental factors may have before deciding on a laboratory or in situ study. Studies conducted at the intended place of performance will be faced with more upfront costs of installing the information system and the difficulty of controlling the experimental conditions in such an environment.

If a system can be placed in its intended surroundings, the use of recording devices and multimedia may reduce the impact of the study on the participants while even increasing the value of the study. For example, when a system is added to the environment where it will be used, video recording or screen/keyboard capturing software can be added to help capture data and evaluate interactions with the system. This may provide very valuable usability data, plus efficiency and effectiveness can also be more easily deduced in this manner. Although an initial "increased awareness" and some changes in behavior can be expected when behaviors are recorded, many people will quickly revert to their customary behavior.

Task or Data

The user task or the stimulus data used in the study is another important element. It is imperative that evaluation tasks are representative of the system's future use. There are several reasons for this. The first is that realistic tasks are necessary if the researcher wants to draw conclusions from the experiment pertaining to the actual work environment. This ensures that the experiment has external validity. Secondly, realistic tasks allow participants to feel more like it is a "real" system and they will behave more like they would working with the "real" system. This increases the external validity of user actions. More realistic tasks will usually also lead to more motivated participants. Finally, it is fairly typical to get very useful comments and advice from participants when they work with realistic data, especially if they are representative users.

Errors and Power

The overall goal of doing a user study is to verify the existence of a causal relationship between the independent variable, the treatment, and the dependent variable, the outcome. In informatics, this treatment involves the use of information technology. If there is an effect of the treatment, the sample of people who received the treatment will differ with regard to the measured outcome from those people who did not receive the treatment. The common method to demonstrate such a relationship is to show a statistically relevant relation between the independent and dependent variable. When the study has enough statistical power, i.e., the ability to show a significance difference between conditions of the independent variable if it exists, the difference will be discovered.

The power of a study is affected by the design of the study, the size of the effect that is being measured, the statistic being used (for example a t-test), the number of participants in the study and also the size of errors that one is willing to accept. These elements are interrelated and can be controlled by the researcher. For example, choosing a within-subjects design may result in more power because of reduced variance. Accepting a higher α (level of significance) will result in more power. However, this will have an effect on how trustworthy the conclusions are, as is described below. In addition, working with more subjects will also have an effect. Usually, having more subjects who participate is better as long as they are representative of the intended users.

Increasing the power of a study and reducing the chance of making an error should be treated differently depending on the type of study being conducted. For example, a pilot study may be conducted to investigate a brand new medical training program that uses virtual patients. In this case, the researcher is interested in finding whether there is a potential effect and whether this line of investigation is worth further consideration. The pilot study serves to guide and fine-tune the research. For example, the researcher could be satisfied with a larger α, such as .10 instead of .05, to indicate significance. In this case, there is a higher chance that the effect will not really be significant. While this is unsuitable for drawing final conclusions, it may be the preferred road to follow in pilot studies where new systems are being considered. Especially in medicine, it would be unfortunate to miss an excellent opportunity, a lead, before it was properly and thoroughly investigated.

To understand how all elements are related and affect the power of a study, it is necessary to understand the difference between Type I and Type II errors. These errors are related to how hypotheses are framed. The following sections therefore explain the different hypotheses and their relation to making errors, the power of a study and the effect size of the treatment.

Hypotheses

The goal of an experiment is to test the causal relationship between two variables: the independent and the dependent variable. The independent variable represents conditions, treatments or levels of treatments that the researcher is interested in. The dependent variable represents the effects of these treatments. This relationship between the two variables is explicitly stated in the research questions and the hypotheses.

When conducting experiments, the research questions are translated into a set of hypotheses: the null hypothesis (H_0) and the alternative hypothesis (H_1). To allow valid conclusions from an experiment, these two hypotheses need to be mutually exclusive and exhaustive. Mutually exclusive means that only one of the two can be accepted as the truth. Exhaustive means that the hypotheses describe all possible scenarios – all options are covered by the two hypotheses. When these conditions are true, then when one hypothesis is rejected, the other one is necessarily true. And so the conclusion of the experiment is clear: one hypothesis or the other is true.

The null hypothesis states that there is no relationship, and the goal of the researcher is to disprove this statement. If this statement can be shown to be incorrect, then the alternative hypothesis has to be true. The hypothesis needs to be stated as such because it is impossible to prove a statement for an entire population; it is impossible to test all members of that population and prove a rule. However, it is possible to disprove a rule if one exception can be found. If the study demonstrated that exception, the null hypothesis has to be rejected and the alternative hypothesis accepted.

For example, assume a study of the preference of nurses for a software product to store electronic health records. After extensive field work, the researchers came up with a design for a new menu system that they believe will lead to different behaviors than the system currently in use. The hypothesis is that the new menu is different from the old menu. To verify this hypothesis, the researchers would have to test their software with every nurse in the world, which is of course a preposterous proposition. Therefore, they conduct an experiment instead and will do a statistical test. They cannot prove their hypothesis is true as explained above. However, they can check whether the reverse (H_0) is false, that is, if the new and old menus are the same. Since both hypotheses are mutually exclusive, only one of the two can be

Table 3.3 Hypothesis statements (*IV* independent variable, *DV* dependent variable)

Specifying mean scores		Specifying the IV-DV relationship
Without directionality	With directionality	
$H_0: X = Y$	$H_0: X > Y$	H_0: no causal relationship between IV and DV
$H_1: X \neq Y$	$H_1: X \leq Y$	H_1: causal relationship between the IV and DV

true. If H_0 cannot be rejected by the experiment, then the researchers would have to go back to the drawing board. However, if the experiment shows that H_0 is false, then the researchers can state that their new menu system is not the same as the old menu system.

The hypothesis can be described in two ways that are equivalent (Table 3.3). Both are used in the literature. The first is to describe the hypothesis as a comparison of means. In this case, the hypotheses are said to describe a relationship between the mean scores for the experimental conditions. For example, a null hypothesis could state that the means for two conditions do not differ. If this null hypothesis is rejected, it can be accepted that the means for the two conditions differ. Or the hypotheses could include directionality.

An alternative way to look at this is by stating the relationship between the independent variable (IV) and the dependent variable (DV). Since the mean scores are intended to be a measurement of the effect of an independent variable, it is equivalent to state the hypotheses as a relationship between the independent and dependent variable. Stating that the means do not differ is the same as stating that there is no relationship between the independent and dependent variable. Since the independent variable is intended to change the scores for the dependent variable, this impact indicates a relationship between the two. If there is no impact, there is no relationship.

For example, assume an experiment to evaluate the online appointment scheduling system for a dentistry office. The system has been designed to reduce the number of changes in appointment times. The underlying assumption is that if people can see all available slots online, they will pick the best one and will be less inclined to change it. The existing appointment method, by phone, is compared with this new one, the online system. The dependent variable is the average number of changes in appointments. The null hypothesis can be stated in two ways. Using the means, it would state: "H_0: mean number of appointment changes with phone system = mean number of appointment changes with online system." Using the alternative method, the null hypothesis would state: "the appointment system does not affect the number of appointments being changed" or "there is no relationship between the appointment system and the number of appointments being changed."

Naturally, no relationship between treatments and outcomes in humans is as black and white as described above. Therefore, statistical tests are used to decide whether to reject the null hypothesis. The test statistics give the probability that the null hypothesis can be correctly rejected, i.e., it is known what the chances are of being wrong by rejecting or being wrong in not rejecting. These are Type I and Type II errors.

Table 3.4 Overview of type I and type II errors

The researcher's decision	Reality: the true situation	
	H_0 is true	H_0 is false
Reject H_0	Type I error	No error
	Probability $= \alpha$	Probability $= 1 - \beta$
Accept H_0	No error	Type II error
	Probability $= 1 - \alpha$	Probability $= \beta$

Type I and Type II Errors

Research questions about the causal relation are rewritten as a null hypothesis and an alternative hypothesis. As explained above, the null hypothesis states that there is no relationship. The goal of most studies is to reject this null hypothesis. Unfortunately, sometimes this hypothesis is rejected while it should not have been rejected. The researcher will assume there is a relationship between the two variables while in reality this is not the case. In other cases, the null hypothesis will not be rejected. The study will have failed to show a relationship and so the null hypothesis stands. But, it is possible that accepting the null hypothesis is incorrect. These two situations, when a decision is made that does not match the reality, are referred to as Type I and Type II errors.

The probability of making a Type I or Type II error describes the correctness of a decision. Table 3.4 shows the overview. To understand these errors, think of the "real world" or reality versus the researcher's decision based on guesses of the state of the real world. When an experiment leads a researcher to reject or accept a hypothesis, this is not necessarily a correct decision. There are many reasons why an experiment leads to one conclusion or the other. Think back to all the examples of bias that affect results. To guard against such errors, it is helpful to understand what the probability is of making such an error. Type I and Type II error probabilities help decide how certain we can be about our decision about the reality based on the outcome of an experiment.

A Type I error, indicated by alpha (α), is also called a *gullibility error* [11]. This error is the probability of rejecting the null hypothesis incorrectly. When this happens, a relationship will be claimed as described in the alternative hypothesis, but it is not true. In most research, the Type I error receives much more attention than the Type II error [11]. The probability of making a Type I error is α or the significance level. If the level of significance, also known as the p-value, is .05, there is a 5% chance that the null hypothesis is incorrectly rejected. Most statistical packages will provide the p-value of the analysis. A commonly accepted maximum threshold for α is 0.05, or a p-value of .05, before a researcher can claim a significant effect. A p-value of .01 or .001 is a much stronger indicator that the null hypothesis can be rejected. A larger p-value, such as 0.1, is not very trustworthy; there is a 10% chance that the null hypothesis is incorrectly rejected (making a Type I error).

A Type II error, indicated by beta (β) and also called a *blindness error* [11], is the probability of accepting the null hypothesis incorrectly. Although this error does not receive as much attention, in medicine the consequences of missing an existing relationship can be enormous. For example, missing a positive effect of new medication would be terrible for the patients. The probability of making a Type II error is β.

Statistical Power

The statistical power of an experiment is its probability of correctly rejecting the null hypothesis. In other words, power is the probability of not making a Type II error (see Eq. 3.21). When a study has sufficient statistical power, it will be able to detect an effect of an independent variable on a dependent variable. However, when there is not enough statistical power, the study will not be able to detect the effect even when it exists. A commonly accepted minimum value for β is 0.80 as the power that an experiment should have.

$$\text{Power} = 1 - \beta \qquad (3.21)$$

There are several interrelated elements that influence statistical power. Some can be controlled by the researcher: the sample size, the study design and even the metrics used. With experiments, the goal is to find a causal relationship between the independent and dependent variable but the strength of such a relationship can be weak or strong. The elements discussed above all relate to each other. Increasing one will have an effect on the others. It is the researcher's job to find a balance that is most suitable for the study.

The effect size will have a large impact. A bigger effect will be easier to measure and will require a less powerful study. However, with more powerful studies, even small effect size can be detected. The effect size is the strength of the relationship in the population between the different conditions of the independent variable and the outcome. It is important to understand that a weak effect size does not mean that the effect is unimportant. This is especially the case in medicine and medical informatics, where even a small effect may have a serious impact on people's lives and quality of life. For example, Leroy et al. evaluated the effect of grammatical changes to text on perceived and actual difficulty of text. There were 86 participants in the study and a within-subjects design was used. A very strong effect was found for perceived difficulty of text. However, the study found no significant effect on actual difficulty of text even though the mean scores on a question-answering task were better with simpler grammar. It is probable that the effect of grammatical changes on understanding is so small that an extremely large group of participants is needed to show a statistically significant effect. Even though this effect seems very small, it is still important: since millions of people make decisions related to their health and healthcare based on what they read [16], improving understanding is very important.

The number of participants (n) in each condition or each combination of conditions also affects the power of an experiment. Think of this number as the number of data points that are available in each condition to measure a treatment. With smaller effect sizes it will take a larger sample of subjects to detect this effect and see a statistically significant difference in the experimental conditions. With a larger effect size, it takes a smaller sample of subjects to detect an effect and see a statistically significant difference in the conditions of the independent variable.

The study design influences its power because it affects how subjects are divided across experimental conditions. When deciding on the number of subjects, it is important not only to think about the total number of subjects, but the number of subjects per condition. For example, when 60 subjects have agreed to participate in a study and the independent variable has six different treatment levels, then a between-subjects design would result in only ten subjects per condition. This would very likely not be enough to detect a significant difference between the conditions, unless the effect size is extremely large.

Although seldom discussed in experimental design and statistics books, there is evidence that the metrics used to measure the dependent variable may also affect the power of a study. Maisiak and Berner [17] compared three types of metrics to measure the impact of diagnostic decision support systems: rank order, all-or-none and appropriateness measures. In their study, physicians were asked to provide a list of possible diagnoses in order of how correct they thought they were. Rank order measures take this order into account and provide a score based on position. All-or-none measures check whether the correct diagnosis is present in the list. Appropriateness measures combine scores associated with each given diagnosis in the list. They found that with the same study design, the same sample and the same dataset, there were still differences in the power of a metric. The rank order metrics showed consistently higher effect sizes. Although this study focused on evaluations of decision support systems, the type of measures are very similar to what is used in search engine studies where ranked results are presented in response to a query.

A final note about power and effect sizes is needed. Understanding these two measures is important because a successful study must have an effect size that is large enough to be detected. However, they are also very useful when comparing studies and interventions. The effect sizes can be compared to evaluate the most effective and efficient interventions. For example, van der Feltz-Cornelis et al. [18] compared treatments of depression in diabetics. Treating depression is important for the patients' general well-being but also because it negatively affects diabetic related outcomes. As part of a meta-analysis including 14 randomized clinical trials, they calculated the effect size of different treatments for depression. They found moderate effects for different treatment options and concluded that psychotherapy combined with self-management education was the preferred treatment because of its large effect.

Robustness of Tests

Statistical tests are based on theoretical distributions. The tests rely on mathematical models. It is only when the underlying assumptions are met that the models hold.

Some tests are considered *robust* against violations of their underlying assumptions. When a test is said to be robust, it means that violating some assumptions has only a limited impact on the probability of making Type I and Type II errors. In other words, the conclusions, such as the need to reject the null hypothesis, are still fairly trustworthy. Note the vague language since the trustworthiness depends on which assumptions are being violated and by how much. For an overview of the effects of violating assumptions, see statistical manuals and ongoing discussions in the literature.

References

1. Kirk RE (1995) Experimental design: procedures for the behavioral sciences, 3rd edn. Brooks/Cole Publishing Company, Pacific Grove
2. Fang J-Q (2005) Medical statistics and computer experiments. World Scientific Publishing Co. Pte. Ltd., Singapore
3. Gravetter FJ, Wallnau LB (2007) Statistics for the behavioral sciences, 7th edn. Thomson Wadsworth, Belmont
4. Raymondo JC (1999) Statistical analysis in the behavioral sciences. McGraw-Hill College, Boston
5. Kurtz NR (1999) Statistical analysis for the social sciences. Social sciences – statistical methods. Allyn & Bacon, Needham Heights
6. Vaughan L (2001) Statistical methods for the information professional: a practical, painless approach to understanding, using, and interpreting statistics. Commercial statistics. Information Today, Inc, New Jersey
7. Ropella KM (2007) Introduction to statistics for biomedical rngineers. synthesis lectures on biomedical engineering. Morgan & Claypool. doi:10.2200/S00095ED1V01Y200708BME014
8. Ross SM (2004) Introduction to probability and statistics for engineers and scientists, 3rd edn. Elsevier, Burlington
9. Riffenburgh RH (1999) Statistics in medicine. Academic, San Diego
10. Lewin IP (1999) Relating statistics and experimental design. Quantitative applications in social sciences. Sage, Thousands Oaks
11. Rosenthal R, Rosnow RL (1991) Essentials of behavioral research: methods and data analysis. McGraw-Hill, Boston
12. Smith CE, Dauz ER, Clements F, Puno FN, Cook D, Doolittle G, Leeds W (2006) Telehealth services to improve nonadherence: a placebo-controlled study. Telemed J E Health 12(3):289–296
13. Heywood C, Beale I (2003) EEG biofeedback vs. placebo treatment for attention-deficit/hyperactivity disorder: a pilot study. J Atten Disord 7(1):43–55
14. Leykin Y, DeRubeis RJ, Gallop R, Amsterdam JD, Shelton RC, Hollon SD (2007) The relation of patients' treatment preferences to outcome in a randomized clinical trial. Behav Ther 38:209–217
15. Sidani S, Miranda J, Epstein D, Fox M (2009) Influence of treatment preferences on validity: a review. Can J Nurs Res 41(4):52–67
16. Baker L, Wagner TH, Signer S, Bundorf MK (2003) Use of the internet and e-mail for health care information: results from a national survey. J Am Med Assoc 289(18):2400–2406
17. Maisiak RS, Berner ES (2000) Comparison of measures to assess change in diagnostic performance due to a decision support system. In: AMIA Fall Symposium. AMIA, pp 532–536
18. Van der Feltz-Cornelis CM, Nuyen J, Stoop C, Chan J, Jacobson AM, Katon W, Snoek F, Sartorius N (2010) Effect of interventions for major depressive disorder and significant depressive symptoms in patients with diabetes mellitus: a systematic review and meta-analysis. Gen Hosp Psychiatry 32:380–395

Between-Subjects Designs

4

Chapter Summary

The previous chapters provided an overview of different types of studies, ranging from naturalist observations to controlled experiments, and how these fit in the software development life cycle. The essential components of a study, such as the hypothesis, the participants and random assignment, were discussed. In addition, the different types of variables were introduced with an illustration of how a design equation incorporates them.

Following these introductions, a first study design principle is explained in detail in this chapter: the *between-subjects* study design [1–4]. This design is also referred to as an *independent measures design*. First the principle behind this design is discussed, namely that there is a separate group of study participants for each experimental condition of a variable. Then, both advantages and disadvantages are described. Three designs that follow the between-subjects principle are worked out. First, the principle can be applied when there is one variable. If this variable has only two conditions, it is most often called an *independent samples design*. When there are more than two conditions, it is called a *completely randomized design*. The between-subjects principle can also be used with two or more independent variables. Then it is called a *completely randomized factorial design*. In each section, the statistical tests best associated with the designs are discussed. These are the independent samples *t*-test and the one- and two-way ANOVA.

The Between-Subjects Principle

When a between-subjects approach is used for the independent variable in a user study, the participants of the study experience only one level of that independent variable. Treatment, level and condition all mean the same, although the word 'condition' is also used to refer to combinations of treatments when there is more than one independent variable. The indexes j and j' (or k and k') will be used to indicate that these are two conditions of the same independent variable.

G. Leroy, *Designing User Studies in Informatics*, Health Informatics,
DOI 10.1007/978-0-85729-622-1_4, © Springer-Verlag London Limited 2011

Each condition will have a different group of participants, and the comparisons of the conditions will be based on differences that are found between the groups of subjects. Following the same approach for all independent variables is the easiest to apply and analyze, but it is not required for a user study. It is possible to combine a between- and within-subjects design in one study. Moreover, a mixed design may sometimes be the better choice. Unfortunately, there are no simple formulas or rules that can be used to decide on the approach to select. The researcher needs to choose the design that best suits the goal of the study and for which there are sufficient resources available to execute the study in a practical manner.

The decision to follow a between-subjects approach needs to be made for each independent variable separately. When the independent variable specifies a personal characteristic, such as the presence of a disease, particular experience or preferences, the between-subjects design is the only possible design. For example, when comparing the use of an image-based texting program by children with autism and children who do not have autism, no child can be assigned to both groups. However, in many other cases the independent variable could be evaluated with a between-subjects, or the alternative, a within-subjects approach, which is discussed in the next chapter. If there is a nuisance variable that can be controlled in this manner, the within-subjects design is a more appropriate choice.

Random assignment of study participants to the different conditions is an essential component of using the between-subjects approach. The randomization process ensures that when subjects are assigned to a treatment, sources of variances will not be systematic. For example, if participants can be of different ages, then randomly assigning each participant to a condition can ensure that one condition does not have an overrepresentation of young participants. True random assignment ensures high internal validity of the experiment and allows the researcher to make conclusions about the experimental treatment with confidence. The age of participants could affect the use of the information system but it is not the main interest of the study, so it would be crucial that the participants of different ages are randomly assigned to each experimental condition. If there were two experimental conditions and one had many more young people, then no confident conclusions could be drawn about the independent variable since age would be a confounded variable.

In medical informatics and medicine, it is customary to demonstrate the effectiveness of the randomization process. It is most often done using chi-square (χ^2) analysis (see Chap. 3). For example, Schroy et al. [5] developed a decision support system (DSS) intended to increase screening for colorectal cancer. Using a between-subjects design, they randomly assigned more than 600 patients to one of three conditions: the basic DSS, the DSS augmented with a module to evaluate personal risk and a control group where participants did not interact with the DSS but received general information instead. The researchers looked at several outcomes, such as patient satisfaction and screening intentions. They used χ^2 analysis to verify that their randomization procedure had been successful. That is, they showed that there were no systematic age differences between the three conditions. If there had been differences, any effects could have been (partly or completely) attributed to this unintentional age gap. Since this was not the case, the difference they found in patient satisfaction with the decision making process could be attributed with more confidence to the treatment levels of the independent variables.

A note of caution is needed. It is easy to get carried away when defining variables. Because a nuisance variable has a systematic effect on the observed scores, it can be confused with potential independent variables. It is important to keep the goal of the study in mind to distinguish between independent variables to be manipulated and the nuisance variables to be controlled. A practical approach to make the distinction is deciding whether a variable is of scientific or business interest. When it is not of interest, it should not be included as an independent variable since it would increase the number of participants required and also the number of main and interaction effects that will not really contribute to the research but make the interpretation of results more difficult.

Advantages

The between-subjects design has several advantages that are related to the validity of the study and the ease with which the study can be conducted. An important first advantage is that there can be no learning between conditions since each participant is exposed to only one experimental condition. This design therefore avoids any contamination of conditions from learning. Moreover, since each condition has its own group of people, more different people will be involved; when all is equal, a larger sample will be a better representation of the population than a smaller sample. Complementary to this is the reduced impact of outliers: their impact will be limited to the one condition and if they need to be removed from the dataset less data will be lost.

There are several additional practical advantages. When participants take part in one condition, the time they spend is usually shorter than if they were to take part in multiple conditions. A shorter time often makes is easier to recruit participants. Many people are more willing to participate in a study that takes 15 minutes versus a study that takes an hour or more. This design is advantageous when participants are on a tight schedule or physically cannot participate in longer studies, due to tiring, stress or other practical problems. Furthermore, because each participant partakes in only one condition, there is more time available per participant and the researcher may choose to use more detailed measures. For example, a full length survey could be used instead of the abbreviated version. It is the researcher's choice to balance the different advantages.

Finally, this approach is usually simpler to design, analyze and organize. Even when there are multiple independent variables or multiple conditions for variables, this design scales up easily.

Disadvantages

As with all experimental designs, there are disadvantages that need to be taken into account. A first disadvantage is related to the expected variance in the sample and the size of the effect. When more different people participate, it is likely that the groups will be less homogeneous and there may very well be more variance in the scores for the outcome variable. If a larger variance exists in response to differences in the sample and the expected effect of the treatments is small, this may make it difficult to detect an effect.

A practical disadvantage is directly related to the number of participants needed for the study. A sufficiently large group of participants has to be recruited for each condition to complete the study. Ideally, the participants are recruited and participate around the same time and under similar conditions to avoid bias. This may become increasingly difficult when there are many independent variables or many experimental conditions. Since each combination requires a different set of participants, the number of required participants may rapidly increase and put a practical limitation on what can be included in the study. The number of participants per condition may also be quite large, for example, thirty per combination, depending on the effect sizes that are being measured. In the medical field, in particular, this may be a significant obstacle since subjects are often patients or clinicians. In other fields, such as education, recruiting many participants may be easier.

One Variable with Two Conditions: Independent Samples Design

The simplest between-subjects design involves one independent variable with two conditions. The study participants are randomly assigned to one of two conditions such that each participant experiences only one condition of the independent variable. Since μ represents the population mean, the notation μ_j is used to represent the mean for the population associated with a specific condition of the independent variable (j) (Eq. 4.1). The complete design equation is the same for two or more conditions and discussed in the next section (Eq. 4.2).

$$\mu_j = \mu + \alpha_j \qquad (4.1)$$

With this design where there are two conditions, it is straightforward to test two types of hypotheses: those that are directional or not. When directional hypotheses or one-sided hypotheses are framed, one mean is hypothesized to be larger than the other. The null and alternate hypotheses look as follows:

$H_0: \mu_j \le \mu_{j'}$ for all j and j'
$H_1: \mu_j > \mu_{j'}$ for at least one j and j'

If no direction between means is hypothesized, the hypotheses are called non-directional or two-sided. The null hypothesis indicates that α_j is hypothesized to be zero. The null and alternate hypotheses look as follows:

$H_0: \mu_j = \mu_{j'}$ for all j and j'
$H_1: \mu_j \ne \mu_{j'}$ for at least one j and j'

Table 4.1 Between-subjects design for one variable with two levels

Information system	
Basic	Deluxe
Y_{11}	Y_{12}
Y_{21}	Y_{22}
...	...
Y_{n1}	Y_{n2}
$\overline{Y}_{.1}$	$\overline{Y}_{.2}$

For example, assume that the independent variable is an information system to track glucose levels (see Table 4.1). It has two versions that the researchers want to compare: the basic and the deluxe version. Both versions provide nutrition and exercise information and glucose tracking options. The basic version has no visualization of data while the deluxe version has visualization. Subjects use either the basic or the deluxe information system, but not both. The outcome variable measures for each subject how well he can control glucose.

Score Y_{11} is the score for the first subject in the first condition (basic system), while score Y_{n1} is the score for the nth subject in the first condition. The mean of the observations for the first group, $\overline{Y}_{.1}$, is compared to the mean for the second group, $\overline{Y}_{.2}$. The average score of the participants in each condition will represent the population mean: μ_j is estimated by $\overline{Y}_{.j}$.

If the two conditions of the independent variable lead to different observations, then the two calculated means will reflect this. However, a statistical test is necessary to conclude that this difference in sample means can be generalized to a difference in population means. This is the basis of inferential statistics.

For a comparison between two groups, the t-test is the most useful and commonly used statistic. The t-test is used to determine whether the two population means represent statistically different populations or not. ANOVA can also be used in this case and would be equivalent, but it is a more general test and is discussed in the next section for variables with more than two conditions. A one-tailed t-test is conducted when the hypothesis includes directionality between the means. A two-tailed t-test is conducted when the hypotheses are non-directional and only a difference in means is hypothesized. If there is no significant effect of the experimental treatment, the researcher cannot reject the null hypothesis. It is important to note that the t-test is limited to comparing only two conditions.

If there are more than two conditions, an ANOVA is more suitable to analyze all differences in one test. If the researcher prefers a t-test or prefers to test all pairs of conditions, he should include a Bonferroni adjustment. A Bonferroni adjustment ensures the risk of committing a Type I error does not increase with multiple tests. It is discussed in Chap. 8.

One Variable with Three or More Conditions: Completely Randomized Design

When the independent variable has three or more levels, the design can be general-ized and is called a *completely randomized design*. The same principles apply with more than two conditions for one independent variable as for two conditions. However, when there are more than two conditions it is more common to test whether there is *any* difference between experimental conditions. Equation 4.2 pro-vides the design formulation for this model. The Y score is the outcome measure that is observed for each participant i in each condition j. It is comprised of three different components. The first is the population mean μ (mu); this is the value around which all observed values will vary. The second is α (alpha), which is due to the independent variable. It is expected to differ for each condition j. Finally, there is ε (epsilon), which is the final portion of the score that is due to error. It is an error that will be different for each individual in every condition ($i(j)$).

$$Y_{ij} = \mu + \alpha_j + \varepsilon_{i(j)} \tag{4.2}$$

The participants need to be randomly assigned to one of the n levels of the inde-pendent variable. The null hypothesis indicates that α_j, the effect of the independent variable, is hypothesized to be zero. This is reflected in the hypothesis statements as follows:

H_0: $\mu_j = \mu_{j'}$ for all j and j'
H_1: $\mu_j \neq \mu_{j'}$ for at least one j and j'

For example, the evaluation of the information system to track blood sugar levels described above could include three conditions for the independent variable. Table 4.2 shows an example with three conditions based on system use: a baseline condition of No Information System, the Basic Information System and the Deluxe Information System. The mean of the observations for the baseline condition with No Information System, $\bar{Y}_{.1}$, is compared to the mean for the Basic Information System, $\bar{Y}_{.2}$, and to the mean of the Deluxe Information System, $\bar{Y}_{.3}$.

When there are more than two conditions for the independent variable, the researcher needs to choose which tests to conduct. An ANOVA is the most appro-priate test in this case. An ANOVA with one independent variable is called a one-way ANOVA. The term "one-way" indicates that there is only one indepen-dent variable.

The ANOVA is a general test to find any significant differences between means. When an ANOVA indicates there are no significant differences, it signifies that there are no significant differences between any of the means. On the other hand, when an ANOVA indicates there are significant differences, it does not tell the researcher which means differ. The largest difference will be significant; however, no informa-tion is given for any of the smaller differences between conditions. Although this may seem obvious from the means themselves, additional post hoc tests are neces-sary to statistically evaluate so that inferences can be made beyond the sample. Post hoc evaluations are discussed in Chap. 8.

Table 4.2 Between-subjects design for one independent variable with three conditions

Information system		
None	Basic	Deluxe
Y_{11}	Y_{12}	Y_{13}
Y_{21}	Y_{22}	Y_{23}
...	...	...
Y_{n1}	Y_{n2}	Y_{n3}
$\overline{Y}_{.1}$	$\overline{Y}_{.2}$	$\overline{Y}_{.3}$

If a researcher prefers to conduct t-tests instead of ANOVA, both directional and non-directional hypotheses can be tested. However, in this case, it is imperative that a Bonferroni adjustment is used. The Bonferroni adjustment avoids increasing the chance of making a Type I error when multiple tests are conducted. It is discussed in Chap. 8.

Two or More Variables: Completely Randomized Factorial Design

The between-subjects design can be applied to studies with more than one independent variable. Such a study design is called a *completely randomized factorial design*. This term refers to the fact that all conditions of two or more variables are included in the design. If there is one independent variable with two treatments and another independent variable with two treatments, there will be four groups of subjects because there are four combinations of treatments. These are called the conditions of the study. When there are more variables and more levels, there will be more experimental conditions. Having more variables does not change the rationale of a between-subjects design: every participant in the study participates in only one condition. Similar to experiments with only one independent variable, it is imperative that subjects are assigned to experimental conditions in random fashion.

As can be seen in the design equation (Eq. 4.3) there are now five components that make up the observed score. The equation reflects that an additional variable contributes to the observed scores. It is assumed here that the treatments are completely crossed. This means that all possible combinations of the independent variables are included in the experiment. The observed score is the score of one individual *i* who participates in the *jk* experimental condition: the combination of condition *j* of the first independent variable with condition *k* of the second independent variable.

Comparable to the previous design equations, the first component is the population grand mean μ which represents the value around which all scores for the different conditions vary. The second and third components are the effect of the first independent variable, represented by α_j, and the effect of the second independent variable, represented by β_k. Both α and β reflect the change in the observed score that can be expected from that respective independent variable. The fourth component is the potential interaction of the two variables; it represents the joint effect of the independent variables with $(\alpha\beta)_{jk}$. This interaction is the specific variation in the score that can only be observed in the *jk* condition. The fifth and last component is the error for each score, $\varepsilon_{i(jk)}$. This is the error that will be different for each individual in each condition. It is the remaining variance that cannot be attributed to any other component.

$$Y_{ijk} = \mu + \alpha_j + \beta_k + (\alpha\beta)_{jk} + \varepsilon_{i(jk)} \tag{4.3}$$

When there are two or more variables, hypotheses can be stated about the individual effects of an independent variable. A significant impact of one variable is called a *main effect*. Each independent variable can have its own main effect. There is a null hypothesis for each independent variable. So, the two null hypotheses state that α_j and β_k will be zero. When written out using means, the null hypotheses look as follows for the first variable:

H_0: $\mu_j = \mu_{j'}$ for all j and j'
H_1: $\mu_j \neq \mu_{j'}$ for at least one j and j'

The hypotheses for the second variable are comparable:

H_0: $\mu_k = \mu_{k'}$ for all k and k'
H_1: $\mu_k \neq \mu_{k'}$ for at least one k and k'

There are also hypotheses that can be stated about the interaction between the variables. If the impact of one variable changes significantly depending on the level of another variable, this is called an *interaction effect*. Depending on the number of independent variables, there can be two-way, three-way or even higher interaction effects. Interaction effects between two variables are easy to interpret. However, higher order interactions become progressively more difficult to interpret.

When there two independent variables, the null hypothesis states that the interaction effect $(\alpha\beta)_{jk}$ is expected to be zero. This means that different levels j and j' of the first independent variable (α) within a level *k* of the second independent variable (β) are considered equal. The difference between the two means is therefore hypothesized to be zero. Similarly, the different levels for that first independent variable (α) are also considered equal in the other levels, *k'*, of the second independent variable (β). The difference between these means also is hypothesized to be zero. Combining these statements into one set of hypotheses can be written as follows:

H_0: $\mu_{jk} - \mu_{j'k} - \mu_{jk'} + \mu_{j'k'} = 0$ for all j, j' and k, k'
H_1: $\mu_{jk} - \mu_{j'k} - \mu_{jk'} + \mu_{j'k'} \neq 0$ for at least one j, j' and k, k'

For example, the information system described above to track blood glucose could also exist in two versions: one version for use on a mobile phone and one version for use on a computer. The researchers randomly assign the study subjects to one of four conditions as shown in Table 4.3. The means for each condition are compared to each other. To test for a main effect of the information system, the mean $\overline{Y}_{.1.}$ is compared with $\overline{Y}_{.2.}$. To test for a main effect of the hardware used, the mean $\overline{Y}_{..1}$ is compared with $\overline{Y}_{..2}$. To test for interactions, the means within each condition are also tested, for example, mean $\overline{Y}_{.11}$ is compared with $\overline{Y}_{.12}$.

Table 4.3 2×2 Between-subjects design for two variables

Hardware		Information system		
		Basic	Deluxe	
	Mobile phone	Y_{111}	Y_{121}	
		...	...	$\overline{Y}_{..1}$
		Y_{n11}	Y_{n21}	
		$\overline{Y}_{.11}$	$\overline{Y}_{.21}$	
	Laptop computer	Y_{112}	Y_{122}	
		...	...	$\overline{Y}_{..2}$
		Y_{n12}	Y_{n22}	
		$\overline{Y}_{.12}$	$\overline{Y}_{.22}$	
		$\overline{Y}_{.1.}$	$\overline{Y}_{.2.}$	

In the example above, with two levels for each independent variable, a significant main effect for an independent variable allows the researcher to conclude that the two levels are significantly different. However, if there are more than two levels for one independent variable, follow-up tests need to be conducted to pinpoint which two conditions are significantly different from each other. Such post hoc tests are discussed in Chap. 8.

When there are two or more variables which each have two or more conditions, an ANOVA is an appropriate test. The ANOVA will allow the researcher to conclude whether there are significant main effects for any of the independent variables. It will also test if there are significant interaction effects between variables. When there are two independent variables, this is called a *two-way ANOVA*. This factorial design can be extended to more variables and more conditions. When there are three independent variables, a three-way ANOVA is conducted, and so on. To specify the number of conditions that are being considered, the notation n x m ANOVA is used to indicate that the first variable has n levels which are completely crossed with the m levels of the second variable. For example, when one independent variable has two conditions that are completely crossed with the three conditions of the second independent variable, this would be noted as a 2x3 ANOVA.

References

1. Kirk RE (1995) Experimental design: procedures for the behavioral sciences, 3rd edn. Brooks/Cole Publishing Company, Pacific Grove
2. Gravetter FJ, Wallnau LB (2007) Statistics for the behavioral sciences, 7th edn. Thomson Wadsworth, Belmont
3. Kurtz NR (1999) Statistical analysis for the social sciences. Social sciences – statistical methods. Allyn & Bacon, Needham Heights

4. Ross SM (2004) Introduction to probability and statistics for engineers and scientists, 3rd edn. Elsevier, Burlington
5. Schroy PC III, Emmons K, Peters E, Glick JT, Robinson PA, Lydotes MA, Mylvanaman S, Evans S, Chaisson C, Pignone M, Prout M, Davidson P, Heeren TC (2010) The impact of a novel computer-based decision aid on shared decision making for colorectal cancer screening: a randomized trial. Medical Decision Making. doi:10.1177/0272989X10369007

Within-Subject Designs

5

Chapter Summary

The first few chapters provided an overview of different types of studies and the different variables that one needs to understand to design a study were explained. The previous chapter focused on a first design principle, the between-subjects design, where each subject participates only in one experimental condition.

This chapter focuses on a second study design principle: the *within-subjects design* [1–4]. It is also called a *dependent measures* or *repeated measures design*. With a within-subjects design, there are two approaches to assigning participants to conditions. With the first, the participants in different conditions are the same people or artifacts. They partake in all experimental conditions. As a result, there are repeated measures conducted for each participant. Alternatively, with the second approach the people or artifacts are different but are treated as the same for the purpose of the study. The participants partake in only one condition but they are matched across conditions based on their similarity to each other with regard to a nuisance variable that is being controlled. Thus, the matched participants in each condition are considered the same for the purpose of the study. These two different approaches to assigning participants do not affect the calculations. Similar to the other designs, the within-subjects design can be used with one or more variables and with variables that have two or more conditions. The statistical tests most commonly performed with this design are the paired samples *t*-test and repeated measures ANOVA.

The Within-Subjects Principle

As in the previous chapter, the terms treatment, level and condition are used interchangeably here and indicate one specific level or combination of levels of the independent variables. The indexes j and j' (k and k' or i and i') are used to indicate that these are two conditions of the same independent variable.

The within-subjects design is used to control error variance or a nuisance variable. When conducting experiments, there may be factors that will affect the results that are not of interest to the researchers. For example, experience levels or training with an information system may differ for individual participants and may affect the results by introducing unwanted variance. Environmental differences, such as the place, time or other circumstances of the study participants, can also play an important role and similarly introduce differences that are not of interest. By matching participants who are similar to each other with respect to this nuisance variable across conditions, much of the error variance can be controlled. This leads to less error variance so that the effect of the independent variable, if it exists, will be more easily found to be significant.

There are several variations on the within-subjects principle. A *repeated measures design* is when the same subjects are observed across all the levels of the independent variable and there are more than two conditions. When there are only two conditions, it is more often called a *paired samples design*. When the subjects partake in all conditions, they serve as their own control. However, the within-subjects principle can also be applied with different participants in different conditions. In this case, the participants will need to be matched to each other across conditions. When participants can form such matched sets with respect to a nuisance variable, this is called *subject matching*. In addition, participants can also be matched based on an already existing and natural grouping or pairing, such as the different children in a family, husband and wife pairs or participants of social groups. It is important that the matching is done for the nuisance variable that the researchers want to control. The matched sets of subjects are then treated as *blocks* in a design.

The within-subjects design is suitable when participating in multiple conditions does not provide any additional effects, the effects of the treatment are short lived, or there is no learning or training during treatments. While this is often difficult to accomplish in the behavioral sciences, it is more common and easily accomplished in informatics where artifacts are often used to test algorithms. In such cases, it is not people who participate but their artifacts. For example, when testing algorithms using blogs, text messages or medical records, these artifacts can be reused in the different experimental conditions. There will be no changes in the artifacts from one condition to the next. Similarly, the treatments will not be different because an artifact has been used in multiple conditions.

Naturally, people can also participate in a within-subjects design in informatics, for example, when testing out different versions of a software product. Random assignment of subjects to conditions is executed differently with this design compared to the between-subjects design. When the study subjects participate in all treatment levels of an independent variable, the subjects need not be randomly assigned but the order of conditions that the subjects participate in will need to be randomized. If the order is randomly decided per subject, then this design is also referred to as a *subjects-by-treatment design*; if the (random) order of treatments is the same for all subjects, this is also referred to as a *subjects-by-trials design* [1]. The randomization is essential. When subjects experience the conditions one after the other, they may become tired, bored, trained or excited while working through the experiment. This will affect the results of the conditions that are conducted later in the sequence. Therefore, the within-subjects design should be reserved for treatments that have no or only a very short term carryover effect.

When the number of conditions is limited, all possible orders of treatments can be included. For example, if there are two conditions for an independent variable, condition A and condition B, then the experiment should use two sequences: A-B and B-A. Random assignment should be used to assign half of the subjects to the first ordering and the other half to the second ordering. When there are three experimental conditions, A, B and C, then the researcher can still easily organize the study so that all possible orderings are included. These orderings are: A-B-C, A-C-B, B-A-C, B-C-A, C-A-B and C-A-B. Again, participants should be randomly assigned to one of the six possible orderings. In this manner, any difference that is found between the experimental conditions will not be due to the ordering. Naturally, the assignment is best balanced so that approximately the same number of participants is assigned to each sequence. When there are more conditions and not every order can be included in the experiment, the order of conditions can be randomized per subject.

The within-subjects design can be used with one or more independent variables. The decision to use a within- or between-subjects approach has to be made per variable. As noted above, it is possible for each variable to have two or more conditions. The statistical tests most commonly performed with a within-subjects design are the paired samples t-test when working with one independent variable with two conditions and the repeated measures ANOVA for the other cases.

Advantages

A major advantage and the main reason for conducting a within-subjects design is that it is extremely well suited to reducing error variance by controlling a nuisance variable. This will increase the likelihood of showing the effect of the independent variable if it exists.

Other advantages are of a practical nature. Fewer participants need to be recruited compared to a between-subjects design. When the users are clinicians or patients, this is a very important advantage. In addition, when the participants need to relocate to participate or when scheduling their time is difficult, this design is easier to organize.

Disadvantages

There are several disadvantages to the design. When the treatment effects carry over to other experimental conditions, the within-subjects design is not appropriate. In addition, other types of learning or carryover effects that are not related to the experimental treatment need to be taken into account [5]. For example, learning about the topic being discussed, learning how to use the computer system or learning more about the experimental procedure itself may have an effect on the results. In addition, people may gain more confidence over time or with multiple sessions and this alone may change their behavior.

The time needed to complete the study may be a disadvantage, especially if the entire study is conducted in one sitting. When participants need to be engaged for a longer time, they may become tired, bored and inattentive. If possible, a break should be included in studies that take a long time to complete to allow people to remain concentrated and motivated. However, when such a break is provided in between treatments, other biases may come into play due to external events that cannot be controlled but may affect the participants. Naturally, the maximum length of a study depends on the participants. For some groups, such as severely ill people, elderly or very young people, shorter time periods are required. The time span should be adjusted to take into account the cognitive disabilities, age and health of the participants.

There are also practical disadvantages. A within-subjects study will take more of the participants' time compared to using a between-subjects design. This will have an effect on recruitment of participants. Fewer people may be available for an extended period of time and fewer will be willing to participate. Retention may also be affected. With longer studies, a higher dropout rate can be expected because people are unwilling or unable to complete the study.

One Variable with Two Conditions: Paired Samples Design

When there is one variable which has conditions in which the subjects can be matched, the design is called a *dependent samples* design. When there are only two conditions, the *t*-test is usually conducted and the analysis is referred to as a *paired samples t*-test. This means that the subjects in the first condition are related to (or identical to) the subjects in the second condition. A comparison of scores is made within each pair of scores. The pairing of subjects is done to control a nuisance variable.

The hypotheses that can be tested with this design are similar to the between-subjects design; however, they take into account that the participants are matched:

$H_0: \mu_j = \mu_{j'}$ for all j and j'
$H_1: \mu_j \neq \mu_{j'}$ for at least one j and j'

In informatics, the subjects of a study can be people or artifacts, i.e., man-made objects. The following shows how artifacts, which are documents in this example, can be used in an experiment. Assume a project where researchers are studying tools to assign a difficulty level to text. As part of this project, the researchers need to assign a gold standard difficulty score to documents. For this, they have conducted a study where subjects read a text and then answer questions by choosing from multiple items. The average number of questions correct for each document provides the researchers with a gold standard of the difficulty level. Now, the researchers' goal is to find an automated approach to measure text difficulty. This

Table 5.1 Within-subjects design for one independent variable with two conditions

	Information system	
	Readability formula	Machine learning
Block 1	Y_{11}	Y_{12}
Block 2	Y_{21}	Y_{22}
...	...	...
Block n	Y_{n1}	Y_{n2}
	$\overline{Y}_{.1}$	$\overline{Y}_{.2}$

automatically assigned difficulty level for each document will be compared against the gold standard.

The most commonly used formulas to assign difficulty scores to documents, the so called readability formulas, are the Flesch Readability Scores and the Flesch-Kincaid Grade Levels. They have been used in many projects to estimate difficulty levels of text [6–12] and use word and sentence length as stand-ins for semantic and syntactic complexity or difficulty [13]. However, the researchers have developed a new machine learning method to score documents and want to compare this new method with the existing readability formula. An experiment is designed to compare both approaches. The researchers calculate how well each approach estimates the difficulty level of the texts in comparison to the gold standard. The same texts are submitted to each system. Table 5.1 shows an overview.

In the example, there are n documents or artifacts that are assigned to both conditions. There is a block for each. Therefore there are n blocks to indicate this matching. The means are calculated in the usual fashion. The analysis will take into account that artifacts were matched. If a t-test is used, the t-value will be calculated using the paired samples approach discussed in Chap. 3.

In this design, an artifact was used for testing. However, the design is not limited to artifacts, but can also be used with people. In that case, each study subject would participate in both conditions of the independent variable. For example, consider an information system to visualize text and help people understand the content. Understanding is measured by providing multiple choice questions and calculating how many were answered correctly. Each participant receives a text and questions without any visualization and another similar text and questions with the visualization system. The order is reversed for half of the participants. This constitutes a paired samples design.

As explained above, the within-subjects design is not limited to participants who experience all conditions. Instead, blocking can be used. Blocking makes it possible to have different people in different conditions. Blocking can be accomplished by matching participants according to their value on a nuisance variable that the researchers want to control. In the example, the reading levels of people could be measured, and people in each condition, with and without visualization, could be matched based on their reading level.

For this design with one independent variable that has two conditions, an ANOVA or a paired samples t-test can be conducted. Although the conclusions that can be drawn would be the same for both tests, the paired samples t-test is more common. In both cases, the analysis needs to take into account that the participants are matched. The t-test does this by conducting an evaluation of differences as was explained in Chap. 3. An ANOVA for such a blocked design, described in the next section, makes this adjustment by reducing the error term by that portion of variance that can be attributed to the blocks. Software packages will take this into account when calculating effects. However, it is the researchers' responsibility to correctly indicate which type of design is used.

One Variable with Three or More Conditions: Randomized Block Design

The randomized block design can be seen as an extension of the dependent samples design. In this design, there are three or more conditions for the independent variable. As with the paired samples design, there is a nuisance variable that is being controlled by blocking. The block can consist of one participant who is treated with all levels of the independent variable or of matched participants. If each participant partakes in all experimental conditions, repeated measures are used. The order of the conditions should be randomized for each individual. Alternatively, if each block consists of participants that are matched to each other then the participants need to be randomly assigned to a condition. Artifacts are also used in these studies in informatics.

How controlling this nuisance variable reduces the error variance is clear from the design equation (Eq. 5.1). The observed score Y_{ij} is comprised of four components. The first component is the population grand mean (μ) around which all scores vary. The second component represents the effect due to the treatment (α_j). The third component represents the effect that can be attributed to the block (π_i). And the final component represents the error variance ($\varepsilon_{i(j)}$), which is that variance that cannot be systematically controlled or assigned to the other components.

$$Y_{ij} = \mu + \alpha_j + \pi_i + \varepsilon_{i(j)} \tag{5.1}$$

In this design, there are two null hypotheses. First, there are hypotheses for the independent variable, as written out below:

$H_0: \mu_{.j} = \mu_{.j'}$ for all j and j'
$H_1: \mu_{.j} \neq \mu_{.j'}$ for at least one j and j'

Second, with this design hypotheses can also be stated about the blocking itself. The researcher would expect this portion to be significant in the statistical tests. Such a significant effect is a good indication that it was worthwhile to conduct the blocking. Note that the subscripts are different from the previous hypotheses and indicate these are differences between blocks, not conditions:

$H_0: \mu_{i.} = \mu_{i'.}$ for all i and i'
$H_1: \mu_{i.} \neq \mu_{i'.}$ for at least one i and i'

Table 5.2 Within-subjects design for one independent variable with three conditions

	Information system			
	Readability formula	Machine learning	Combined system	
Block 1	Y_{11}	Y_{12}	Y_{13}	$\overline{Y}_{1.}$
Block 2	Y_{21}	Y_{22}	Y_{23}	$\overline{Y}_{2.}$
...	...	...	...	...
Block n	Y_{n1}	Y_{n2}	Y_{n3}	$\overline{Y}_{n.}$
	$\overline{Y}_{.1}$	$\overline{Y}_{.2}$	$\overline{Y}_{.3}$	

For example, assume that the Flesch-Kincaid Readability formula and the new machine learning algorithm (mentioned earlier) did not perform as well in the first experiments as the researchers had hoped. However, the researchers are convinced that they will surpass their previous results by combining both approaches. An augmented system is developed that uses a voting scheme to combine the readability formulas and the machine learning approach. The researchers decide to test this approach and conduct a new experiment. As is shown in Table 5.2, there is one independent variable, the system, which has three levels: readability formulas, machine learning and the combined approach.

In this example, each document is now evaluated using the three different approaches. The average score for each condition is compared using a repeated measures ANOVA. An ANOVA can compare the three levels with each other as part of one test. With paired samples t-tests, three tests would have to be conducted to test each pair of conditions, increasing the chance of making a Type I error.

In general, when there are three or more conditions and one independent variable, a one-way ANOVA is the most appropriate statistical test and the researcher would select a repeated measures ANOVA. As was explained in Chap. 3, the F-test compares different variances. The variance described by the numerator is due to the sum of the experimental effect and the error variance. The variance described by the denominator is due to the error variance only. By applying this blocked design, more variance can be systematically assigned to the blocks and removed from the error variance. The variance in the numerator is therefore due to the sum of the experimental effect, the blocks and the remaining error variance. The variance in the denominator is the remaining error variance. By reducing the denominator, the F-value will be larger and so there will be a better chance that it exceeds the critical value.

Two or More Variables: Randomized Block Factorial Design

The within-subjects principle can be applied to studies with two or more independent variables that each have two or more conditions. As with the simpler designs, the participants are blocked based on a relevant characteristic that the researchers want to control. Assignment to the different conditions is done in the same manner as with one independent variable. If participants are matched based on a characteristic, then they should be assigned to treatment levels in random fashion within their block. Alternatively, the order of the conditions should be randomized if the participants are exposed to all conditions.

The design equation reflects that there are two independent variables and a nuisance variable (Eq. 5.2). Obviously, more independent variables can be included and the design equation would be adjusted accordingly. This example equation for two independent variables and a block variable shows how the observed value Y_{ijk} is comprised of seven components. The first component is the population mean, μ, around which all values vary. The second and the third components, α_j and β_k, represent the treatment effects of the two independent variables. The fourth component, $(\alpha\beta)_{jk}$, represents the possible interaction or joint effect of the independent variables. The fifth component, π_i, represents the effect of the nuisance variable that is being controlled; while the sixth component, $(\alpha\beta\pi)_{jki}$, represents the joint effect of the experimental and nuisance conditions. The last component, ε_{ijk}, is the remaining error variance that cannot be attributed to the other parts.

$$Y_{ijk} = \mu + \alpha_j + \beta_k + (\alpha\beta)_{jk} + \pi_i + (\alpha\beta\pi)_{jki} + \varepsilon_{ijk} \qquad (5.2)$$

Similar to the completely randomized factorial design, which includes two or more independent variables, the hypotheses cover the effects for each independent variable and their interactions. The null hypothesis for the first independent variable states that α_j will be zero, while the null hypothesis for the second independent variable states that β_k will be zero. Written out using the means, the hypotheses look as follows for the first variable:

$H_0: \mu_j = \mu_{j'}$ for all j and j'
$H_1: \mu_j \neq \mu_{j'}$ for at least one j and j'

The hypotheses for the second variable are comparable:

$H_0: \mu_k = \mu_{k'}$ for all k and k'
$H_1: \mu_k \neq \mu_{k'}$ for at least one k and k'

In addition, a null hypothesis is stated for the interaction effects between the independent variables. Depending on the number of independent variables, there can be two-way, three-way or even higher interaction effects. Interaction effects between two variables are easy to interpret. However, higher order interactions become progressively more difficult to interpret.

When there are two independent variables, the null hypothesis states that the interaction effect $(\alpha\beta)_{jk}$ is expected to be zero. This means that different levels j and j' of the first independent variable (α) within a level k of the second independent variable (β) are considered equal. The difference between the two means is therefore hypothesized to be zero. In addition, the different levels j and j' of the first independent variable are also considered equal in any other level k of the second independent variable. The difference between these means also is hypothesized to

Table 5.3 Within-subjects design for two independent variables with each two conditions

	Information system				
	Standalone		With human correction		
	Readability formula	Machine learning	Readability formula	Machine learning	
Block 1	Y_{111}	Y_{112}	Y_{121}	Y_{122}	$\overline{Y}_{1..}$
Block 2	Y_{211}	Y_{212}	Y_{221}	Y_{222}	$\overline{Y}_{2..}$
–	...	...	...	...	...
Block n	Y_{n11}	Y_{n12}	Y_{n21}	Y_{n22}	$\overline{Y}_{3..}$
	$\overline{Y}_{.11}$	$\overline{Y}_{.12}$	$\overline{Y}_{.21}$	$\overline{Y}_{.22}$	

be zero. Combining these statements into one set of hypotheses can be written as follows:

$$H_0: \mu_{jk} - \mu_{j'k} - \mu_{jk'} + \mu_{j'k'} = 0 \qquad \text{for all j, j' and k, k'}$$
$$H_1: \mu_{jk} - \mu_{j'k} - \mu_{jk'} + \mu_{j'k'} \neq 0 \qquad \text{for all j, j' and k, k'}$$

The previous hypotheses covered effects of the independent variables. However, since this design uses blocking, the effects of blocking can also be evaluated. It should be noted that in the design presented here, it is assumed that the interaction effects of the independent variables with the block are zero (this is called an *additive model*). If this is assumed not to be the case, additional interaction effects between each independent variable and the blocks need to be added to the design equation.[1] For the current design, the hypotheses for the nuisance variable can be stated as follows:

$$H_0: \mu_{i.} = \mu_{i'.} \qquad \text{for all i and i'}$$
$$H_1: \mu_{i.} \neq \mu_{i'.} \qquad \text{for at least one i and i'}$$

Table 5.3 shows an overview for the example. Assume that the information system introduced above to evaluate text difficulty uses either the Flesch-Kincaid Readability formula or the new machine learning algorithm. The approach is a first independent variable. However, the system can be used in a standalone version or it can be used by a human expert, for example, a librarian who adjusts the outcome of the system. The researchers are interested in finding out how this affects the usefulness of the system and therefore include a second independent variable: standalone versus human correction. The blocking remains the same. Comparable documents, the artifacts, are submitted to all four experimental conditions.

The researchers calculate the average score in each condition and compare these averages using a two-way ANOVA (a 2×2 ANOVA). Note that for this artifact, the

---

[1] For the non-additive model, the two interactions $(\alpha\pi)_{ji}$ and $(\beta\pi)_{ki}$ should be added to the design equation (5.2).

order of the conditions does not matter for the system's evaluation but needs to be randomized for the human. The text will not appear differently because it has been evaluated before; there is no risk of carryover effects. If humans were evaluated instead of artifacts, then the order of treatments would have to be randomized for each participant.

In general, an ANOVA is the most appropriate test to conduct for this design. A repeated measures ANOVA would be conducted with two independent variables. By indicating that the scores are blocked across all conditions when running the statistical analysis, the F-values will be calculated using an adjusted numerator and denominator with a lower error variance. If there are significant effects, this design will give the researchers a better chance of finding them.

References

1. Kirk RE (1995) Experimental design: procedures for the behavioral sciences, 3rd edn. Brooks/Cole Publishing Company, Pacific Grove
2. Gravetter FJ, Wallnau LB (2007) Statistics for the behavioral sciences, 3rd edn. Thomson Wadsworth, Belmont
3. Kurtz NR (1999) Statistical analysis for the social sciences. Social sciences – statistical methods. Allyn & Bacon, Needham Heights
4. Ross SM (2004) Introduction to probability and statistics for engineers and scientists, 3rd edn. Elsevier, Burlington
5. Friedman CP, Wyatt JC (2000) Evaluation methods in medical informatics. Springer-Verlag, New York
6. Berland GK, Elliott MN, Morales LS, Algazy JI, Kravitz RL, Broder MS, Kanouse DE, Muñoz JA, Puyol J-A, Lara M, Watkins KE, Yang H, McGlynn EA (2001) Health information on the Internet: accessibility, quality, and readability in English and Spanish. JAMA 285:2612–2621
7. D'Alessandro D, Kingsley P, Johnson-West J (2001) The readability of pediatric patient education materials on the World Wide Web. Arch Pediatr Adolesc Med 155:807–812
8. Root J, Stableford S (1999) Easy-to-read consumer communications: a missing link in Medicaid managed care. J Health Polit Policy Law 24:1–26
9. Bluman E, Foley R, Chiodo C (2009) Readability of the patient education section of the AOFAS Website. Foot Ankle Int 30(4):287–291
10. Cheung W, Pond G, Heslegrave R, Enright K, Potanina L, Siu L (2009) The contents and readability of informed consent forms for oncology clinical trials. Am J Clin Oncol Oct 30. [Epub ahead of print]
11. Greywoode J, Bluman E, Spiegel J, Boon M (2009) Readability analysis of patient information on the American Academy of Otolaryngology-Head and Neck Surgery Website. Otolaryngol Head Neck Surg 141(5):555–558
12. Bernstam EV, Shelton DM, Walji M, Meric-Bernstam F (2005) Instruments to assess the quality of health information on the World Wide Web: what can our patients actually use? Int J Med Inform 74(1):13–19
13. DuBay WH (2004) The principles of readability. Impact information: http://www.impact-information.com/impactinfo/readability02.pdf. Last accessed on January 20, 2011

Advanced Designs

6

Chapter Summary

Previous chapters discussed the between-subjects and within-subjects design principles and associated experimental designs. This chapter discusses variants using the between- or within-subjects designs as building blocks. First, it is shown how they can be combined with each other in a study and how, depending on the number of variables, several different combinations are possible. A few examples are provided in this section. This is followed by a description of how two nuisance variables can be controlled in a study with one independent variable by using a Latin Square Design. Finally, Model I and Model II specifications are explained in the last section. Since most researchers today use software packages to calculate variance where options can easily be checked or unchecked, it has become deceptively easy to conduct analyses. However, understanding the differences can help the researcher conduct better studies and draw the correct conclusions.

Note that this chapter does not provide an exhaustive list of possible study designs. Many others may be of interest, such as the various hierarchical designs where treatments are nested or those using one or more covariates. However, by understanding the basic designs discussed here, the reader can consult and understand the advanced statistical books and then design and conduct such studies accordingly.

Between- and Within-Subjects Design

As was discussed in the previous two chapters, each variable in the user study needs to be considered by itself to decide whether to follow a within- or between-subjects design. When more variables are being evaluated, it is not always possible, nor is it necessary or optimal, to use only one principle for all variables. Some variables may be better tested with a within-subjects approach and others with a between-subjects approach. Both approaches can be successfully mixed in a study.

G. Leroy, *Designing User Studies in Informatics*, Health Informatics,
DOI 10.1007/978-0-85729-622-1_6, © Springer-Verlag London Limited 2011

Studies that combine one within-subjects variable with one between-subjects variable are fairly common in informatics. Often, the within-subjects approach is used to establish a baseline, for example, a measurement before and after training with an information system. The between-subjects variable frequently is the variable that describes the different versions of an information system. Naturally, variations are possible. With careful consideration of the time needed to complete a condition and taking into account possible carryover or other potential biases, it is often possible to conduct more comprehensive evaluations by including within-subjects variables without increasing the number of participants or the variance drastically. Two examples are discussed next.

Miyahira et al. [1] used one within- and one between-subjects variable, each with two levels, in their study. They compared two display types, flat screen and immersive virtual reality, to provide therapy to treat anger disorders. One phase of their study focused on eliciting anger reactions using one of the two displays. Of their 60 participants, 30 were assigned by random selection to the flat screen condition and the other 30 to the immersive virtual reality condition. Each participant was tested pre- and post-treatment using an anger expression inventory. Independent samples t-tests were conducted to compare the anger reaction between the two display types. This comparison showed a significant advantage of using the virtual reality interface. A dependent samples t-test was also conducted on the pre- and post-scores which showed a significant effect in the virtual reality display group. In this study the dependent samples t-test confirmed that the immersive virtual reality was a stronger instigator of anger expressions since it led to a significant effect with the immersive reality but not with the flat screen display.

Saadawi et al. [2] used a more complex design. They worked with pathology residents to evaluate a computer-based, intelligent tutoring system that provided automated feedback on actions taken by the students. There were different versions of the system that needed to be compared. The researchers evaluated the computer system with a within- and between-subjects mixed approach. They compared three tests: first the pathology residents were tested without using a system, then while using a baseline tutoring system, and finally while using one of two versions of an improved version of the tutoring system. Half of the residents worked with the improved version that used supplementary metacognitive support, while the other half worked with the same system without the extra support. A within-subjects comparison was possible for the entire group between the condition without a system and with the baseline system. Within-subjects comparisons were also possible for each subgroup between the baseline system and the improved system they used. Finally, a between-subjects comparison was possible between the two improved versions. They found immediate feedback to be beneficial.

Although the statistical analysis becomes somewhat more complicated, this should not be a reason to avoid a mixed design. Most statistical packages available today are user friendly and allow researchers to specify the type of design used for each variable. The packages take care of making the correct calculations.

Blocking Two Nuisance Variables: Latin Square Design

Chapter 5 discussed how blocking can be used with a within-subjects design to control a nuisance variable. The *Latin Square design* is an extension of this design that makes it possible to control two nuisance variables. Keep in mind that the Latin Square design is different from a study with two independent variables that are being controlled. With the latter, a two-way ANOVA would be conducted. The Latin Square design controls two nuisance variables in addition to evaluating the impact of one independent variable. These nuisance variables are known to affect the results but are not of interest in solving the research problem. However, since they contribute to variability within the groups when not controlled, it is better to control them. This design also assumes that there are no interactions between variables.

The term Latin Square originates from an ancient puzzle game. Today's Sudoku players will recognize the rules of the game. A Latin Square consists of n rows and n columns. The goal of the puzzle is to put a symbol in each cell so that no row and no column have repeated symbols. There are as many symbols as there are rows or columns. Table 6.1 shows an example of a Latin Square design. Note that there are alternative orders in which the square could be filled out to fulfill the requirements. For example, the first row could contain the BCDA sequence which would affect all other cells in the square. A Latin Square is called a *standard Latin Square* when the first row and column are ordered. If the symbols are letters, the ordering is alphabetical; if the symbols are numbers, the ordering is numerical. The Latin Square in Table 6.1 is a standard Latin Square.

To apply the Latin Square design, the independent variable must have as many levels as both the nuisance variables. Table 6.2 shows an example of a design of an experiment with one independent variable (A) that has four conditions (A1, A2, A3, A4) and two nuisance variables. The nuisance variables are controlled using a standard Latin Square. Each treatment appears four times in the square: once for each combination of the two nuisance variables, and the first row and first column are ordered.

For example, assume a persuasive anti-smoking information system that has four levels of persuasion (A1, A2, A3, A4) to help people quit smoking. Each level uses increasingly more concrete images and forceful persuasion techniques, ranging from simple text messaging to showing images of the lungs of diseased smokers. The outcome being measured is the reduction in number of cigarettes smoked after 3 months. There are two nuisance variables to be controlled. The first nuisance variable is the number of cigarettes smoked per day at the beginning of the trial. Some participants may smoke very few cigarettes while others may smoke more than a pack a day. It can be expected that their starting amount of cigarettes per day will affect the outcome. The second nuisance variable is the number of years smoking. Some participants may have recently started smoking, while others may have been smoking for years. It is also expected that the length of their smoking habit, measured in years, will affect the outcome.

Table 6.2 shows how each version of the information system is tested with each type of smoker. To control the first nuisance variable, the researchers distinguish

Table 6.1 Example of a 4×4 Latin Square

A	B	C	D
B	C	D	A
C	D	A	B
D	A	B	C

Table 6.2 Example of a 4×4 Latin Square experimental design

Independent variable: A1-A4 – persuasive anti-smoking system	Nuisance variable 1: number of cigarettes				
		<5	5–15	15–25	25+
Nuisance variable 2: years of smoking	<1	A1	A2	A3	A4
	1–5	A2	A3	A4	A1
	5–10	A3	A4	A1	A2
	10+	A4	A1	A2	A3

between four levels of smoking: fewer than 5 cigarettes, 5–15 cigarettes, 15–25 cigarettes and more than 25 cigarettes per day at the beginning of the trial. To control the second nuisance variable, the researchers distinguish between four levels of years of smoking: less than 1 year, 1–5 years, 5–10 years, more than 10 years. The Latin Square design makes it possible to measure the effect of each version of the system while controlling for the other sources of variances. For example, to measure the number of cigarettes using system version A1, the four cells containing measures of A1 need to be combined. It is also possible to test the effect of those nuisance variables. For example, differences between light smokers (<5 cigarettes) and moderate smokers (5–15 cigarettes) could be measured.

The design equation (Eq. 6.1) shows how error variance is controlled with this design. By reducing the error variance, the study has more power and will be more likely to show an effect if it exists. Because more variance is controlled, the remaining error variance term becomes smaller. With an F-test this can be seen from the formulas where the denominator in the F-value calculation, the error variance, decreases. A larger F-value will more easily surpass the critical value and show a significant effect.

The observed score, Y_{ijkl}, is comprised of six components. The first component is the grand mean, μ, which is the overall value around which all values vary. The second component is the treatment effect, α_j, which is constant for each observation for a given treatment. The third and fourth components, β_k and γ_l, represent the effects of the nuisance variables. Finally, the fifth and sixth components represent error variance: the fifth component, $\varepsilon_{i(jkl)}$, is any error variance for an individual in each cell, while the sixth component, ε_{jkl}, represents all remaining error variance not yet captured.

$$Y_{ijkl} = \mu + \alpha_j + \beta_k + \gamma_1 + \varepsilon_{i(jkl)} + \varepsilon_{jkl} \tag{6.1}$$

An ANOVA is the most appropriate method for analyzing these effects. The researchers will focus on finding an effect of the treatment (α, see A1-A4 in

Table 6.2) with the analysis. If such an effect is found, the researcher is assured it cannot be due to either of the two nuisance variables, since each level of each nuisance variable is equally represented in each treatment condition. However, if an effect is found for one or both of the nuisance variables, the researcher knows that this effect is only due to the nuisance variables and not to the treatment because every treatment appears in each level of both nuisance variables.

The Latin Square design is very helpful when the order of conditions may affect the outcome. The order itself can be seen as a nuisance variable. When this is the case, the researcher should ensure that the different possible orderings of the conditions are equally represented in the design. Applying the Latin Square design gives the researcher a systematic approach to counterbalancing the ordering of the treatments. For example, Staggers and Kobus [3] compared a graphical and a text based user interface with a group of nurses. All participating nurses completed several tasks with each system. The researchers used a Latin Square design to counterbalance the tasks and interface types. They found higher satisfaction, faster completion times and fewer errors with the graphical version of the system.

In practice, Latin Square designs are most appropriate when there are five or more conditions in the independent variable resulting in a 5×5, or higher, Latin Square. This results in higher degrees of freedom than with smaller designs and more precise F-values [4, 5]. More extensive versions of the Latin Square design exist, as well as different ways of mixing it with a randomized block design. For example, the *Graeco-Latin Square* makes it possible to control three nuisance variables. The *Hyper-Graeco-Latin Square* takes the design a step further with an additional nuisance variable. A *crossover design* has features of both the Latin Square design and the randomized block design. The reader is referred to statistical manuals for these designs [4–6] and statistical software manuals for guidance on how to submit the data.

Fixed and Random Effects Models

When defining a statistical model for a completely randomized design using a one-way ANOVA, the researcher can determine whether a Model I (fixed) or Model II (random) specification needs to be used for the study calculations.

The difference between a *fixed* and *random effects model* specification refers to a different interpretation given to the independent variable. A *fixed effects model* or *Model I* specification assumes that the levels of the independent variable considered in the experiment are the only ones of interest to the researchers. This is in contrast to a *random effects model* or a *Model II specification* where it is assumed that the levels of the independent variable specified in the experiment are only a subset of the different possible levels of the independent variable. The subset used in the experiment is considered a random sample of these possible levels.

The design equation is the same for the fixed and random effects models. For example, assuming a completely randomized design, the design equation can be shown as in Eq. 6.2. The observed score Y_{ij} is composed of three components: the grand mean μ around which all values will vary, the effect of the independent variable α_j and the remaining error variance, $\varepsilon_{i(j)}$.

$$Y_{ij} = \mu + \alpha_j + \varepsilon_{i(j)} \tag{6.2}$$

The nature of the levels of the independent variable is assumed to be different in the two models. As a result, the conclusions that can be made also are different. For example, when evaluating two versions of a system, a fixed effects model would be appropriate. With this model, the conclusions that can be drawn are limited to these two conditions, the two versions of the system. However, assume an example study where a researcher takes a different approach and evaluates one information system with different groups of subjects. The researcher chooses three groups that differ in age because she suspects this will affect the usage of the system. The chosen age groups are far enough apart to cover a range of ages. She chooses three age groups: people between 20 and 30 years old, between 40 and 50 years old, and between 60 and 70 years old. These three groups are a sample of all existing groups and in this case, a random effects model would be more appropriate.

The fixed and random effects models can be mixed in an analysis of variance, with one or more variables considered fixed and one or more variables considered random. A different model specification will lead to different calculations being conducted for the F-value.

References

1. Miyahira SD, Folen RA, Stetz M, Rizzo A, Kawazaki MM (2010) Use of immersive virtual reality for treating anger. Stud Health Technol Inform 154:82–86
2. Saadawi GME, Azevedo R, Castine M, Payne V, Medvedeva O, Tseytlin E, Legowsk E, Jukic D, Crowley RS (2010) Factors affecting feeling-of-knowing in a medical intelligent tutoring system: the role of immediate feedback as a metacognitive scaffold. Adv Health Sci Educatoin Theory Pract 15(1):9–30
3. Staggers N, Kobus D (2000) Comparing response time, errors, and satisfaction between text-based and graphical user interfaces during nursing order tasks. J Am Med Inform Assoc 7(2):164–176
4. Kirk RE (1995) Experimental design: procedures for the behavioral sciences, 3rd edn. Brooks/Cole Publishing Company, Pacific Grove
5. Rosenthal R, Rosnow RL (1991) Essentials of behavioral research: methods and data analysis. McGraw-Hill, Boston
6. Fang J-Q (2005) Medical statistics and computer experiments. World Scientific Publishing Co. Pte. Ltd., Singapore

Part II

Practical Tips

Understanding Main and Interaction Effects

7

Chapter Summary

The first part of this book described the principles underlying experimental design and the associated statistical analyses. The second part focuses on the practical aspects of conducting experiments. Understanding the underlying principles is essential to conduct a successful study. In addition it is helpful to know how to put those principles into practice in an efficient manner that is respectful and beneficial to the different stakeholders.

This chapter focuses on recognizing different effects in the results and using the correct terminology to describe them. Both main and interaction effects are systematically introduced for studies with one, two and three independent variables. Main effects can be found in studies with one or more independent variables. Interaction effects can be found in studies with two or more independent variables. When one finds statistically significant main and interaction effects, a visual inspection of the data can be very helpful in understanding these effects and especially in understanding their implications. Reading the numbers from the output of a statistical package is not enough. One needs to be able to interpret them in the context of the experiment and translate them to broader situations. It is important to know that the list in this chapter is by no means an exhaustive list of possible effects. It is also important to understand that a visual inspection is insufficient to verify whether main and interaction effects are significant. Statistical analysis is needed.

One Independent Variable

In informatics, many experiments are conducted using one independent variable. This is usually an information system, an algorithm or an interface. Three types of studies are common: studies where a new system is compared against a baseline, studies where different versions of a system are compared with each other and a combination of these two. When the new system is compared against a baseline, the baseline can be an existing but different system or it can be the 'lack of' a system, in other words,

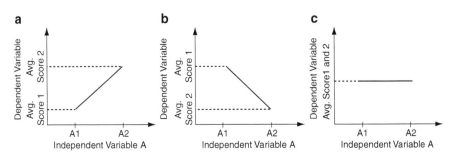

Fig. 7.1 Example of effects for one independent variable with two conditions

a missing system. For example, Ljótsson [1] compared a new Internet-based therapy for irritable bowel syndrome with an online forum. When different versions of a system are tested, these versions often differ on one feature, such as complexity, number of features provided or expense. The approach is the same for all these studies: there is one independent variable with multiple (two or more) levels.

When an experiment has one independent variable, only a main effect can be found. In this case, the effect is usually just referred to as 'an effect'. If there are only two conditions, then a significant effect means that there is a significant statistical difference between the two conditions. If there are more than two conditions, a significant main effect indicates that there is at least one pair of conditions that is significantly different. However, it is possible that there are more pairs of conditions that are significantly different. Post hoc tests need to be conducted to identify which pairs are significantly different. The types of statistical tests suitable for post hoc analyses are outlined in Chap. 8.

To demonstrate effects, a line graph is used to display the data in this chapter. However, bar charts and other variations are used and acceptable. Bar charts may show more clearly that the conditions of the independent variable are discrete. However, line graphs are used in this chapter because they show more clearly the differences between average scores of conditions, especially when there are two or more variables. The figures are idealized to best show the different effects.

Two Conditions

The simplest study design has one independent variable with two conditions. This design simplifies analysis because finding a significant effect means that the two experimental conditions differ and no post hoc analysis is necessary. Such effects can take different forms. Figure 7.1 shows examples. On the x-axis are the conditions of the independent variable. On the y-axis are the average scores for these conditions. Lines are used to connect them to demonstrate how the averages differ between conditions.

Figure 7.1a and b show example significant effects. The figures by themselves cannot show which results are significant, but they are meant to help interpret the results from the statistical analysis. In the case of an independent variable with only two conditions, a significant result from a *t*-test or ANOVA that indicates a significant difference lets the researcher conclude which average is significantly higher. Figure 7.1a shows how there is a significantly higher score in Condition 2 than in Condition 1; Fig. 7.1b shows the reverse with a higher score in Condition 1 than Condition 2. Figure 7.1c shows how the means of the two conditions are nearly equal and there is no effect of the independent variable. Even if the means differ slightly, the effect may not be significant.

When the effect of the independent variable is evaluated on multiple dependent variables, it is common to find a main effect for one dependent variable but not for another. This lack of an effect can be as important as any significant effect. For example, in medical informatics it is often desirable to have a new system that is at least as good as the old system for one measure but better than the old system for another measure. For example, this is the case when information technology is shown to be as good as existing therapies for clinical outcomes but significantly better for other variables, such as satisfaction, cost or convenience.

With new technology, a straightforward comparison between the technology and the baseline condition without technology can provide very valuable insights for further system development. For example, Baur [2] compared two methods to conduct orthognathic evaluations: the customary clinical exam and the same exam using telemedicine. They found significant differences in measurements, for example, the malar bone width tended to be measured as larger with the telemedicine approach. The authors concluded that the current telemedicine application is therefore appropriate for preliminary examinations. Differences in measurements will need to be taken into account with further development and improvement of the technology.

Especially when artifacts and not subjects are used, study designs with one variable may be a convenient, simple and efficient approach. For example, clinical documentation practices have relied for decades on dictation or writing, which allows errors to creep into the text. The use of a graphical user interface with menus and templates has been thought to improve quality of documentation by reducing incorrect information and enforcing standards. The U.S. Department of Veterans Affairs (VA) developed a GUI-based system that uses protocol-based templates for VA disability exams which are implemented using a point and click format. Fielstein et al. [3] compared the quality of the clinical documentation for the original and the new documentation tools. The study used artifacts: the clinical exams completed for the VA Compensation and Pension Examination Program (CPEP) conducted during 2 months in 2005. Quality indicators were used to score each exam, and the researcher found that the quality scores were significantly higher for the exams conducted using the new approach.

Three Conditions

When an independent variable has three or more conditions, a main effect can be found for many different types of outcomes. When there are more than three conditions the number of combinations that can result in a significant main effect also

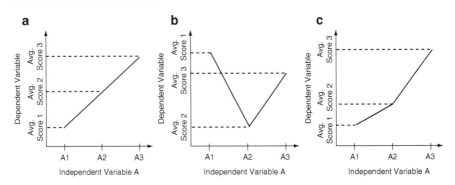

Fig. 7.2 Example of main effects for one independent variable with three conditions

increases quickly. In this case, it is important to conduct post hoc analysis to verify which pairs of conditions differ significantly. Figure 7.2 shows three fictitious examples for a study with one independent variable that has three conditions. Assuming that there was a significant main effect, the researcher knows that the largest difference that exists between two conditions will be significantly different. However, no other conclusions can be made without post hoc analysis.

Figure 7.2a shows an example of the three conditions having increasingly higher average scores. If an ANOVA indicates there is a main effect for this variable, then it is possible that the differences between all pairs of conditions (1 and 2; 2 and 3; 1 and 3) are significant. However, it is also possible that only the difference between Condition 1 and 3 is significant.

Figure 7.2b shows a very different example. Here, Condition 2 resulted in a low average score but both Conditions 1 and 3 resulted in a high average score. A significant main effect means that at least the largest difference between a pair of conditions is significant. In this example, this is the difference between Condition 1 and 2. However, post hoc analysis will be needed to verify whether the differences between Condition 2 and 3 and possibly between Condition 1 and 3 are significant.

Figure 7.2c shows an outcome that is similar to example A, where the researcher can conclude that the difference between Condition 1 and 3 is significant. However, in example C the difference between Condition 1 and 2 is much smaller than the difference between Condition 2 and 3. It is possible that both of these differences are not significant or that only the difference between Condition 2 and 3 is also significant.

Studies with three or more conditions for an independent variable are common in informatics. For example, in 1996 Murphy et al. [4] evaluated the effects of Iliad, a diagnostic consultation system designed to help teach differential diagnosing in internal medicine. In a study with 33 subjects who had different levels of training (12 students, 12 residents and 9 attending physicians), the researchers evaluated the effect of Iliad on diagnosing. They found several main effects of using Iliad. For example, one main effect was the different impact Iliad had on participants with different levels of training. Post hoc analysis showed that students added more diagnoses from the Iliad list than residents did and also more than attending physicians did. In a more recent study with multiple levels of a system, Bigman et al. [5] used a one-way ANOVA to evaluate the effectiveness of 5 versions of educational materials about the human papillomavirus (HPV) vaccine on perceived vaccine effectiveness and opinions about the vaccine. They found significant main effects for the type of text used. Follow-up analysis showed how positive framing led to higher perceived effectiveness of the vaccine.

Lack of Effects

When there are two conditions of an independent variable and no effect is found where it was expected, it is possible that the design of the study contributed to this lack of effect. When the conditions of the independent variable are not chosen appropriately, effects may be missed. How to avoid this is discussed in Chap. 15. This current section is limited to showing two examples that may not result in a statistically significant effect.

Figure 7.3a shows a fictitious example of a study conducted with an independent variable with four conditions. As can be seen from the figure, the differences between Condition 1 and 2 and between Condition 3 and 4 are almost negligible. It is the difference between Condition 2 and 3 that is significant. When a researcher does not choose the conditions appropriately, for example, not extreme enough, then only Condition 1 and 2 might have been included in the experiment. This would lead to the erroneous conclusion that there was not an effect.

Figure 7.3b shows a related example. If nothing were known about the study, it would seem clear that there is an increase in scores from one condition to the next. A significant main effect would be expected for this independent variable. However, if these differences are small, a fact not always obvious from graphs, there may be no effect at all. In this case, it is often valuable to investigate whether there is a significant correlation between the outcome variable and levels of the independent variable. Finding a significant correlation would be a good indication that the independent variable may affect the outcome under different circumstances. For example, it may be an indication that the experimental conditions were not sufficiently different; or another possibility is that the sample size was not sufficiently large and there was insufficient statistical power. A more detailed explanation and examples are provided in Chap. 15.

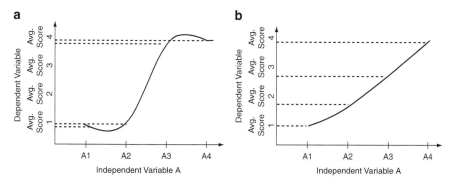

Fig. 7.3 Examples of effects with one independent variable with multiple conditions

Two Independent Variables

Many studies in informatics are more complicated and include multiple independent variables. This is because in studies with human participants, multiple independent variables are often of interest and are expected to influence the results. Moreover, since recruiting participants is time consuming and takes significant effort, many researchers prefer to combine the testing of multiple variables in one study.

In informatics, the most common independent variable is the information system with different conditions. When the information system is the main unit of analysis, additional independent variables are often included because different results can be expected in different environments, for example, rural hospitals versus university hospitals (first independent variable) and with different user groups, for example, novice users or expert users (second independent variable). In other cases, a detailed analysis of an algorithm or system is undertaken and the different versions of the system are systematically evaluated for different types of data. For example, an evaluation can look at a rule-based versus a machine learning approach (first independent variable) and the type of input, complex or simple (second independent variable).

When an experiment contains two independent variables, both main effects and interaction effects can exist. They can appear in many different variations. The statistical results will indicate for which variable a main effect exists and for which variables an interaction effect exists. The figures by themselves are insufficient to make conclusions about main and interaction effects; however, the visual representation is valuable in helping interpret the results. Similar to studies with only one independent variable and more than two conditions, a two-way or three-way (or higher) ANOVA is an omnibus test that does not specify which conditions of an independent variable are significantly different. Post hoc analysis needs to be used to pinpoint all significant differences.

Main Effects

In general, a main effect exists when the effect of one variable is the same regardless of the level of the other variable(s). There can be a main effect for every independent variable in a study, and figures will be very helpful in correctly interpreting the results. Figure 7.4 demonstrates a few commonly found main effects in studies with two independent variables. To make the effect as clear as possible, the figures are idealized. The first independent variable (A) and its conditions are placed on the X-axis. The second independent variable (B) and its conditions can be distinguished with different symbols, lines or labels. The y-axis displays the average score for the dependent variable in the experimental conditions.

Figure 7.4a shows a main effect for Variable A and no effect of Variable B. The average score in Condition A2 is higher than Condition A1 regardless of the scores of Conditions B1 and B2. This indicates the main effect of Variable A. The averages for B1 and B2 are the same regardless of Condition A. This shows the lack of effect of Variable B.

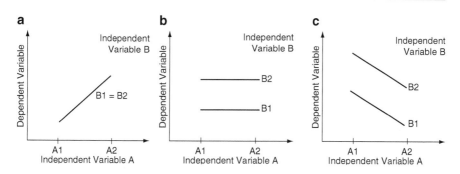

Fig. 7.4 Examples of main effects with two independent variables

Figure 7.4b shows a main effect for Variable B but no effect for Variable A. The average score is higher in Condition B2 compared to Condition B1 regardless of the score of Conditions A1 and A2. This signifies the main effect of Variable B. The average scores for A do not differ in the two conditions, which signifies the lack of an effect.

Figure 7.4c demonstrates two main effects. The average score is higher in Condition A1 than in A2 regardless of the level of B. In addition, the average score is higher in Condition B2 than in B1 regardless of the level of A. This indicates a main effect of Variable A and a main effect of Variable B.

Main effects are commonly found. For example, a few years ago Rickert et al. [6] evaluated the impact of gender and instruction method (computer-assisted instruction, physician-delivered, or no instruction) on knowledge of alcohol and marijuana using a two-way ANOVA. They measured knowledge about and satisfaction with the approach. For knowledge about the topic, they found two main effects similar to the effects shown in Fig. 7.4c. Subjects in intervention groups were more knowledgeable and males were more knowledgeable than females. The authors also report an interaction effect (discussed below), but this was for a different measure; it was for satisfaction with the approach. Males were more satisfied with the computer-assisted instruction.

Interaction Effects

An interaction effect exists between two independent variables when the effect of the one independent variable depends on the level of the other independent variable. Interaction effects can therefore appear in two-way, three-way and more complicated n-way ANOVAs. Interaction effects can exist without main effects. However, having multiple variables or having multiple main effects does not always lead to interaction effects. Figure 7.5 demonstrates commonly found interactions between two variables without any main effects of those variables.

Figure 7.5a shows one type of interaction between independent variables A and B. The graph can be read in two manners. The average score is much higher in

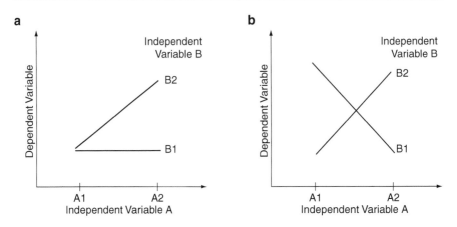

Fig. 7.5 Examples of interaction effects with two independent variables

Condition A2 than in Condition A1 but only under B2. In contrast, the average scores of A1 and A2 do not differ under B1. This change in effect of one variable (A) depending on the level of another variable (B) is what makes an interaction effect. The same interaction effect can also be read as follows by focusing on Variable B. The scores for the two conditions of Variable B (B1 and B2) differ only in Condition A2; in Condition A1, the average score for B1 is the same as for B2.

Figure 7.5b shows a different type of interaction effect. Again, the scores for Variable A differ depending on the condition of B. However, the scores increase from Condition A1 to A2 under Condition B2 but decrease under Condition B1. As with the previous interaction effect, this graph can also be read from the standpoint of Variable B. The scores for Variable B decrease from Condition B1 to Condition B2 under Condition A1. On the other hand, the scores for Variable B increase from Condition B1 to Condition B2 under Condition A2.

Interaction effects are commonly found, especially when there are more than two conditions for one of the independent variables. For example, Belucci [7] worked with patients with schizophrenia and cognitive impairments and tested a system for computer-assisted cognitive rehabilitation. The researcher tested the interaction of two independent variables: the time (pre- and post-evaluations) and the treatment (computer-assisted versus control condition). They valuated the effects and found that only the experimental group performed better on the post-evaluation compared to the pre-evaluation for a variety of cognitive measures.

Main and Interaction Effects

With two or more independent variables, main effects and interaction effects can both be found in one study. For a study with two independent variables, it is possible to have a main effect of one or both independent variables combined with an inter-

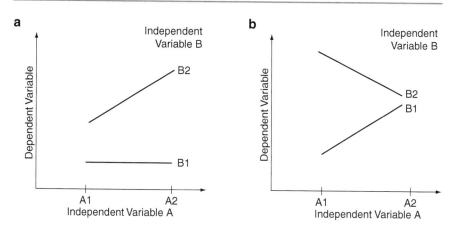

Fig. 7.6 Examples of main and interaction effects with two independent variables

action effect between the two variables. Figure 7.6 demonstrates two frequently found combinations for a study with two variables. Naturally, there exist other possible combinations. Especially when there are more than two independent variables, more different combinations may be found.

Figure 7.6a shows a main effect for Variable B and an interaction between Variable A and B. The main effect of Variable B is based on the scores for Condition B2 which are always higher than those for Condition B1 regardless of the condition of Variable A. In addition, there is an interaction effect between the two variables. Under Condition B1, the scores do not differ between A1 and A2. On the graph, this is clear from the 'B1' line that remains flat. However, under Condition B2, the scores increase from Condition A1 to Condition A2. On the graph, this can be seen by the upward slope of line 'B2'. In other words, the difference in scores from one Condition A1 to A2 depends on the condition of Variable B.

Figure 7.6b shows another example of main and an interaction effects. This is again a main effect of Variable B: the scores in Condition B2 are always higher than the scores in Condition B1, regardless of the condition of A. However, the differences between the two conditions of Variable A are also different in the two conditions of Variable B. Under Condition B1, there is an increase in scores from A1 to A2. Under Condition B2, there is a decrease in scores from A1 to A2.

Cruz et al. [8] conducted an evaluation of new information technology and reported both a main and interaction effect. They conducted a two-way ANOVA to evaluate the effect of camera resolution and bandwidth on the recognition of facial affect in the context of mental health services. Sixty medical students participated and were randomized to one of four conditions. They were asked to identify four facial affects presented via videotape. The researcher found an interaction effect: different camera resolutions and bandwidth combinations had different effects on facial recognition. They also found a main effect of camera resolution on facial recognition.

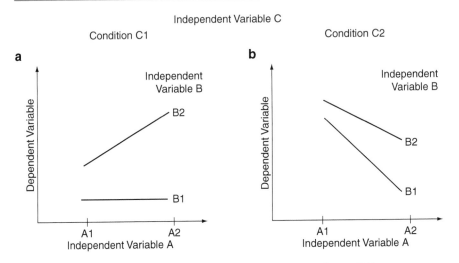

Fig. 7.7 Examples of main and interaction effects with three independent variables

Three or More Independent Variables

Most studies in informatics will have two or fewer independent variables. This does not mean that it is impossible or unacceptable to conduct a study with more independent variables. However, multiple variables will require more complex statistical analysis and may become harder to execute. In addition, when there are more than two independent variables, more types of effects can exist. There can be main effects for every independent variable and interaction effects between any two independent variables. In addition, there are also higher-order interactions that become possible. For example, an interaction between three independent variables exists when the interaction between two variables differs based on the conditions of a third. Interactions that involve more variables become increasingly difficult to interpret.

Since so many different possibilities exist, only one example is demonstrated below. Figure 7.7 shows an illustration of three independent variables and a three-way interaction. This figure shows a main effect of Variable B: the scores are always higher for Condition B2 than B1 regardless of the condition of Variable A or Variable C. There is also an interaction between Variables A and B similar to the interactions discussed above. Finally, there is an interaction between the three variables: the interaction between Variables A and B is different under Condition C1 than under Condition C2.

As noted above, studies with more than two variables are less common in informatics. Carlbring et al. [9] provide an example of a study with three independent variables. Their main goal was to compare the state of relaxation as the result of the first independent variable, the approach, which had three levels: a computer application to administer relaxation, a therapist-guided approach or a control condition where subjects browsed the Internet. The researchers also evaluate the effect of two more independent variables: gender and time period. The effect was measured with both objective and subjective measures of relaxation. Galvanic skin response was the objective measure, while a survey was used for the subjective measure. Although no three-way interactions were found, the study illustrates how multiple types of interactions can be found. The authors report several two-way interactions; a few examples for the objective measure are an interaction between the time period and approach and an interaction for the time period and gender. They also report a main effect for group for the subjective measure, with the control group feeling less relaxed.

With an increasing number of variables and conditions, many more different combinations of effects can be found. The omnibus F-test shows where main and interaction effects can be found. It is the researcher's task to follow up on these effects with post hoc analysis.

References

1. Ljótsson B, Falk L, Vesterlund A, Hedman E, Lindfors P, Rück C, Hursti T, Andréewitch S, Jansson L, Lindefor N, Andersson G (2010) Internet-delivered exposure and mindfulness based therapy for irritable bowel syndrome – a randomized controlled trial. Behav Res Ther 48(6): 531–539. doi:doi:doi:10.1016/j.brat.2010.03.003
2. Baur DA, Pusateri AE, Kudryk VL, Jordan R, Ringgold C, Vandre R, Baker T (1998) Accuracy of orthognathic evaluation using telemedicine technology. Telemed J 4(2):153–160
3. Fielstein EM, Brown SH, McBrine CS, Clark TK, Hardenbrook SP, Speroff T (2006) The effect of standardized, computer-guided templates on quality of VA disability exams. In: AMIA annual fall symposium, Washington DC, 11–15 November 2006, pp 249–253
4. Murphy GC, Friedman CP, Elstein AS, Wolf FM, Miller T, Miller JG (1996) The influence of a decision support system on the differential diagnosis of medical practitioners at three levels of training. In: AMIA annual fall symposium, 1996, pp 219–223
5. Bigman CA, Cappella JN, Hornik RC (2010) Effective or ineffective: attribute framing and the human papilloma virus (HPV) vaccine. Patient Educ Couns 81(Suppl):S70–76
6. Rickert VI, Graham CJ, Fisher R, Gottlieb A (1993) A comparison of methods for alcohol and marijuana anticipatory guidance with adolescents. J Adolesc Health 14(3):225–230
7. Bellucci DM (2000) The effectiveness of computer-assisted cognitive rehabilitation for patients with chronic mental illness. The New School University, New York
8. Cruz M, Cruz RF, Krupinski EA, Lopez AM, McNeeley RM, Weinstein RS (2004) Effect of camera resolution and bandwidth on facial affect recognition. Telemed J E-Health 10(3):392–402
9. Carlbring P, Björnstjerna E, Bergström AF, Waara J, Andersson G (2007) Applied relaxation: an experimental analogue study of therapist vs. computer administration. Comput Hum Behav 23:2–10

Conducting Multiple Comparisons

8

Chapter Summary

Previous chapters described how to choose and combine different independent variables and their conditions. When there are more than two conditions for these variables, additional statistical analysis is needed to verify which differences between conditions are significant. This chapter describes the steps that need to be taken when there are more than two conditions that are being compared with follow-up statistical tests.

Both t-tests and ANOVA can be used to conduct multiple comparisons. When t-tests are conducted, each test indicates whether a difference between two conditions is significant. However, each test carries its own risk. As a result, making multiple comparisons increases the chance of making a Type I Error - where a null hypothesis is incorrectly rejected. To avoid increasing the overall chance of making a Type I Error, a Bonferroni adjustment should be made. On the other hand, when ANOVA is conducted the omnibus F-test shows main and interaction effects. When there are more than two conditions, these significant effects by themselves do not indicate which pairs of conditions differ from each other and follow-up analysis is needed. With ANOVA, the additional analysis consists of post hoc comparisons to pinpoint the conditions where the differences are significant. The Tukey Honestly Significant Difference (HSD) Test is appropriate in this case.

Types of Comparisons

When there are three or more conditions for one independent variable, there are three or more means that can be compared against each other. For example, when there are two versions of an information system that are being compared with a baseline, there are three pair-wise comparisons that can be made: between the baseline and each version of the information system and between the two versions of the information system. Conducting such a set of tests is referred to as conducting a *family of tests*.

G. Leroy, *Designing User Studies in Informatics*, Health Informatics,
DOI 10.1007/978-0-85729-622-1_8, © Springer-Verlag London Limited 2011

Pair-wise comparisons refer to tests that compare two means with each other. When they are all related to the same independent variables, they can be considered a family of pair-wise comparisons. When there are k different conditions for an independent variable, the number of possible pair-wise comparisons is calculated as shown in Eq. 8.1:

$$Pair - wise\ Comparisons = \frac{k(k-1)}{2}\ \text{for k conditions} \qquad (8.1)$$

Post hoc analysis is not limited to pair-wise comparison. Other types of contrasts between means can be tested. For example, contrasts can be used to test for linear, quadratic or cubic trends in data. The reader is referred to statistical handbooks for a detailed explanation of these more advanced analyses [1–3].

In addition to the tests described in this chapter, *Scheffé's test* is also commonly found in the literature and available in most standard statistical software packages. It is a post hoc test suitable for multiple comparisons where the risk of a Type I Error needs to be managed. *Scheffé's* is a very conservative test that is also based on variance. It compares the mean squares for the between condition comparison (in the numerator) with the mean squares of the overall ANOVA (in the denominator). This means that the same critical value is used for each individual test as for the overall ANOVA. As a result the test is less powerful than the *Tukey HSD Test* which is discussed below. However, it is not limited to pair-wise comparisons and so is an excellent tool to compare other types of contrasts when there are three or more means.

Bonferroni Procedure for Multiple t-Tests

With a family of tests, it should be taken into account that each test by itself carries the risk of making a Type I Error. Recall that a Type I Error is made when the null hypothesis is incorrectly rejected and the alternative hypothesis is incorrectly accepted. When α is the probability of rejecting the null hypothesis incorrectly with one *t*-test, this probability will increase when multiple t-tests are conducted. A Bonferroni adjustment needs to be made to avoid increasing the risk of making a Type I Error for the family of tests.

The *Bonferroni procedure* is also called the *Dunn test* [4]. It was first worked out by Dunn [5] who relied on the Bonferroni or Boole inequality [3] principle. Dunn used the inequality to show for t-tests that the *family-wise* or *experiment-wise* Type I Error, the overall error associated with all tests for an experiment, is smaller than the sum of all the individual errors. The principle also applies to other statistics and is not limited to the *t*-test. Using this principle, a maximum acceptable error probability can be chosen for a family of tests.

The *Bonferroni adjustment* in hypothesis testing refers to the adjustment of α for each individual *t*-test so that the probability for all tests combined, the family-wise

α, is set to the maximum probability of making a Type I Error that the researcher is willing to accept. To ensure that the overall risk does not increase, the risk of making a Type I Error for each individual test has to be smaller than the overall risk. The most common adjustment is to treat all individual tests equally and divide α by the number of tests. The formula to divide the overall risk is shown in Eq. 8.2 for a family of tests that are considered equally important.

$$\alpha_{adjusted} = \frac{\alpha}{k} \text{ for k equally important pair-wise comparisons} \qquad (8.2)$$

When all comparisons are considered equally important, the overall risk will be divided over those individual tests in equal portions. For example, if a researcher wants to compare the basic and expert version of a new decision support system (DSS) with a baseline condition, there are three conditions of the independent variable: Baseline, Basic DSS, and Expert DSS. If the researcher will only accept an overall probability of 5% of making a Type I Error, each individual t-test needs to use a smaller probability. There are three comparisons that will be made: No DSS - Basic DSS, No DSS – Expert DSS, and Basic DSS – Expert DSS. With the overall acceptable risk of committing a Type I Error at 5% ($\alpha=0.05$), the level of each test should be set at one-third of the overall risk or 1.67% ($\alpha=0.0167$).

The adjustment can also take into account that some tests are more important than others and use a weighting scheme to adjust the risks. Equation 8.3 shows how each test can be weighted by importance; the weight (W) reflects the importance of a test and is chosen by the researchers. Even so, keep in mind that the combined α value should be equal to the overall risk that was assigned to the study. For formulas and a detailed explanation, see Rosenthal and Rosnow [1]. For example, if there are three tests, they could be weighted as follows: 40%, 40% and 20% (weights of 40, 40 and 20, and a total sum of 100).

$$\alpha_{adjusted} = \frac{W_j}{\sum_1^k W_j} \cdot \alpha \text{ with j indicating a specific pair-wise comparison} \qquad (8.3)$$

When reporting the results, researchers can report whether the null hypothesis can be rejected or not for the adjusted α. This is done in the customary manner by first adjusting the value for α, acquiring the associated critical value for t and evaluating whether the calculated value for t for the experiment is larger than this critical value. If it is larger, the null hypothesis can be rejected.

Since it is increasingly common to report the exact p-values and not only whether they were smaller than a predefined level, the adjusted p-value can also be calculated and reported. Similarly to adjusting α, the p-value needs to be adjusted for the number of tests that are conducted. The formula for equally weighted tests is shown in Eq. 8.4:

$$p_{adjusted} = p.k \text{ for k equally important pair-wise comparisons} \qquad (8.4)$$

When not all tests are weighted equally, the value for p is adjusted as shown in Eq. 8.5:

$$p_{adjusted} = \frac{\sum_1^n W_j}{W_j} \cdot p \text{ with } j \text{ indicating a specific pair-wise comparison} \quad (8.5)$$

With the increasing availability of statistical software that is easy to use and has many options filled in with default values, requiring less statistical knowledge of the users, conducting statistical tests has become almost effortless. As a result, the software is increasingly used to test a variety of hypotheses. It is also used in new ways. Some new information systems are designed specifically to take large sets of data and search (or 'mine') for significant relationships. In both cases, researchers need to be aware that adjustments are necessary to avoid increasing the chance of making a Type I Error. For example, Jin et al. [6] developed such software which helps discover biologists' DNA motifs. The researchers include Bonferroni adjustments in their system for their tests. This is critical since it is especially important to be aware of and protected from the increased risk of errors with this type of application.

Post Hoc Comparisons with ANOVA: Tukey HSD Test

When conducting multiple comparisons, a distinction needs to be made between *a priori* and *posteriori* comparisons. *A priori comparisons* are planned comparisons between means that the researchers intended to carry out even before conducting the omnibus ANOVA. It is argued that the risk of a Type I Error is not inflated with such planned comparisons and that different tests should be conducted. For a detailed discussion and description of a suitable a priori test such as the *Student Multiple t- test*, D*unnette's*, D*unn's* or *Dunn-Šidák's Multiple Comparison* tests, see Kirk [3]. In contrast, *posteriori* or *post hoc comparisons* are also called 'data snooping' and they are conducted after an ANOVA indicated that there were some significant differences.

In this section, only post hoc comparisons are discussed with the assumption that additional measures need to be taken to avoid inflating the risk of making a Type I Error. Several different tests exist. The *Tukey Honestly Significant Difference (HSD) Test* is discussed here because it is among the most popular post hoc tests in many disciplines. The Tukey HSD Test is suitable for pair-wise comparisons with two-directional null hypotheses.

When an experiment is conducted with three or more levels for the independent variable, it is appropriate to conduct an ANOVA. Recall from Chap. 3 that ANOVA uses variance, a measure of variability, to examine the differences between means. The F-test is conducted to check whether the variance between the groups is larger than the variance within groups. The analysis is referred to as an omnibus test because all different means are compared using one test. A significant effect does not let the researcher pinpoint individual significant differences between pairs of means. For this, post hoc comparisons need to be conducted. Similar to the t-tests discussed above, each individual post hoc test carries the risk of a Type I Error where the null hypothesis would be incorrectly rejected. This risk increases when multiple tests are conducted. Post hoc analysis is a formal approach to conduct such multiple tests without increasing the risk of a Type I Error.

By conducting a Tukey HSD Test, the researcher can discover which individual pairs of means differ significantly from each other. The principle is the same as for analyses discussed in previous chapters. The difference between two means is compared to a critical value. If the calculated difference is larger than the critical value, then the difference is considered to be statistically significant. Statistical software packages will refer to this adjusted critical value when conducting post hoc tests.

The calculations needed for the Tukey HSD Test are based on ANOVA and use the variance already calculated as part of the analysis. The critical value is called the Honestly Significant Difference and is calculated as shown in Eq. 8.6. There are three elements in the equation. The first component is the within-group variance represented by the Mean Squares within the group. The second component is represented by the symbol q and stands for the Studentized Range Statistic. Its value is pre-calculated, similar to t and F critical values, and is available from published tables [3] or from statistical software. The value is based on degrees of freedom, the number of comparisons that are being made and the family-wise α that is set by the researcher. The third component is the sample size which is represented by n and is considered equal for all samples. The Tukey HSD Test is suitable for comparisons between conditions that have equal sample sizes. When the sample sizes are unequal, the *Tukey-Kramer Test* can be conducted.

$$HSD = q \sqrt{\frac{MS_{Within}}{n}} \qquad (8.6)$$

Conducting post hoc analysis provides valuable additional information to researchers that cannot be gained from a review of the descriptive data. Similar to all statistical analyses discussed in this book, it is part of the statistical inference process. Choosing the most appropriate tests and being aware of the chance of making errors is an essential part of the inference process. Executing this process correctly and accounting for the aggregate chance of error across multiple tests can substantially increase the value of the results.

References

1. Rosenthal R, Rosnow RL (1991) Essentials of behavioral research: methods and data analysis. McGraw-Hill, Boston
2. Fang J-Q (2005) Medical statistics and computer experiments. World Scientific Publishing Co. Pte. Ltd., Singapore
3. Kirk RE (1995) Experimental design: procedures for the behavioral sciences, 3rd edn. Brooks/Cole Publishing Company, Pacific Grove

4. Gravetter FJ, Wallnau LB (2007) Statistics for the behavioral sciences, 7th edn. Thomson Wadsworth, Belmont
5. Dunn OJ (1961) Multiple comparisons among means. J Am Stat Assoc 56(293):52–64
6. Jin VX, Apostolos J, Nagisetty NSVR, Farnham PJ (2009) W-ChIPMotifs: a web application tool for De Novo Motif discovery from ChIP-based high-throughput data. Bioinformatics 25(23):3191–3193. doi:10.1093/bioinformatics/btp570

Gold Standard and User Evaluations

9

Chapter Summary

In informatics, information systems are being evaluated for their impact on users and the intended environment. This evaluation can be done in two manners which can complement each other. Evaluations can use a gold standard, constructed before the start of the study, to compare against the output of an information system. Evaluations also can be conducted with intended users to assess their actions or interactions with the system. The difference between the two lies in how the input is provided to the information system and consequently how the output is evaluated.

The first approach is to provide input in a systematic, non-interactive manner and compare the output against a predefined gold standard. Although artifacts are usually the units of analysis in such studies, the outcome of user interaction can also be compared against a gold standard. A second approach is for the information system to be evaluated during its interaction with the intended users. In this case, people are the 'subjects' in the study. Each evaluation type has advantages and disadvantages. In many cases, working with a gold standard evaluation is optimal in the early development phases of a system, while working with representative users is optimal in later stages where all components are integrated and the system is more mature. Often, using both approaches is advisable to ensure that enough data points are collected to allow valid comparisons between systems. Gold standards are especially useful to test individual algorithms. In contrast, systems that require interaction with users, such as a decision support system, are very difficult to test with a gold standard.

Gold Standards

A gold standard in an evaluation is a reference point that represents the ideal solution to a problem and is created in advance of a study. In theory, this is the solution that has no errors. These solutions can take on different forms. For example, gold

G. Leroy, *Designing User Studies in Informatics*, Health Informatics,
DOI 10.1007/978-0-85729-622-1_9, © Springer-Verlag London Limited 2011

standards can consist of diagnostic images and their correct diagnoses; they can consist of search engine queries, a collection of available documents, and the lists of documents that are relevant to each query; and they can consist of tagged text and many other types of input/output combinations. Ideally, the gold standard is optimized for efficient processing and evaluation; for example, evaluations can be automated if the gold standard is machine readable. For example, Denny et al. [1] used a gold standard in their evaluation of information extraction algorithms for medical records.

Once a gold standard is available, different versions of algorithms or system outcomes can be compared against it. It is crucial that the gold standard contains the correct solution that does not change for the duration of the evaluation. The same gold standard can be used to compare different versions of an information system because there is no learning effect from one trial to the next for an algorithm. A system will not respond differently to a case because it has been processed in a previous trial. Naturally, researchers cannot adjust their algorithm or system during the evaluation to better suit the gold standard. This would tune the system to that particular gold standard and the study would lead to an overly positive, and dishonest, evaluation of the system.

The type of gold standard and how it was created may affect the outcome of the study because it will affect how representative the standard is. When the gold standard is based on definitive tests, for example, biopsies, the creation of the gold standard is straightforward and objective. However, in many cases, the gold standard is not such a black-and-white outcome. For example, a collection of 'relevant' articles in response to a search query or a collection of 'optimal' educational pamphlets for sharing with patients is not as easily created. One or more people, usually experts, will need to collaborate on creating such a gold standard. Understanding how it was created will help the researcher be aware of its shortcomings. Four types of gold standards can be distinguished:

1. *Gold standards created by using information* that provides an objective, correct solution based on definitive tests. Such standards are usually used to evaluate systems that are being developed to deliver the given answer without the benefit of the definitive test. A common example is the classification of images of masses as benign or not. Algorithms can be trained to distinguish between the two based on non-invasive data with the ultimate goal of providing a correct solution and bypassing invasive tests. The gold standard will include the results from the definitive tests conducted, such as biopsies.

2. *Gold standards created by a single individual.* While this is an efficient method to create a gold standard, care should be taken that the standard is not limited to representing one individual's opinion, ideas or solutions. This would limit the external validity of any evaluation using this standard.

3. *Gold standards created by a group of individuals.* The group usually will consist of experts or representative users. Standards created in this manner provide better external validity because they are more representative of future users. However, one should be aware of the decision process used in the group. When group members do not agree on an outcome, a decision still has to be made. The

process used to come to agreement may introduce random variation into the standard. For example, the solution with the most votes in the group can be chosen for the standard or the solution advocated by the most prestigious team member. *Cohen's Kappa* is a measure used to describe the agreement between individuals and could be used to evaluate the standard itself. A gold standard becomes less of a standard when there is little agreement.

4. *Gold standards created by computer.* Because creating a gold standard takes time, effort and resources, some researchers prefer to create a gold standard by computer. Such a gold standard can be expected to be very systematic, unless some random error was introduced. Studies that compare information systems or algorithms compared against such a systematic gold standard can overestimate the system being evaluated. Moreover, the gold standard may not be entirely representative of how humans would approach the task.

A gold standard should contain a variety of representative cases that the system is expected to handle. There should be a sufficient number of cases - at minimum enough cases for a statistical comparison between different experimental conditions. A generally accepted rule of thumb is that 30 data points are needed per experimental condition. Ideally, however, more data points are needed so that researchers can make a random selection from the entire set for each separate evaluation. Note that with machine learning, very large gold standards are required: usually a few (hundred) thousand examples. A subset of the cases is used to train the algorithms - the training dataset, and the remaining subset of cases is used to test the algorithm after training - the test dataset. See the discussion on n-fold cross-validation in Chap. 2.

Advantages

One advantage of using a gold standard is that *fewer people are involved* than when using study participants. No subjects need to be recruited, which makes it easier to manage the study, and it is faster to conduct if the gold standard is already available. It also facilitates the Institutional Review Board (IRB) process in some cases. For example, when experts compile a gold standard, no IRB approval is needed. However, if the gold standard consists of patient records or other information that includes personal identification information, the researcher should check with their IRB or funders whether approval is required.

A second set of advantages stems from the longevity and permanence of a gold standard. Once it has been created and when it is sufficiently large, it can be *reused for different evaluations*. For example, gold standards are used to compare and contrast algorithms as part of computing competitions [2]. When a gold standard is created, often only a subset of its data is needed for a particular evaluation. When enough 'new' examples remain, the gold standard can be used for a system that has been improved from the version that was first evaluated. The gold standard can also be used with *different versions of a system*. Since there is no learning between information systems, a within-subjects design can often be used for the study and the same input data can be used in all different conditions of the experiment. Finally, because a gold standard is a standalone dataset, it can also be *shared among different researchers*. Chapter 12 lists resources, including some example gold standards.

Finally, some evaluations may be especially well suited to using gold standards because they are readily available or can be created fairly easily. This is true in medicine, where medical records show different levels of information leading to a final conclusion. The records contain the definitive tests and disease outcomes which are essential for a good gold standard.

Disadvantages

Although a gold standard may be very efficient, there are disadvantages associated with its use. A first disadvantage is the *extra work* that is involved in creating it. It will require additional resources beyond those available for the system development: it takes a significant amount of time to create a gold standard, requires the availability of experts and is an additional process that needs to be managed, organized and executed. Especially when multiple experts are required to collaborate on a standard, this process should be formalized. At a minimum, how decisions are reached when experts disagree should be documented.

When a gold standard is created by people and not based on definitive tests, *biases and inconsistencies* may weaken it. Unsystematic variance or variance unrelated to the standard itself may become an inherent part of the standard. For example, when a team of experts collaborates on defining a standard, they may not all agree on what the best solution is. Some type of decision process will be adopted, for example, a vote or follow-the-leader decision, to decide on the final labeling in the gold standard. This information usually is not available in the gold standard itself and so it will be extremely difficult for any information systems to take into account, leading to more errors during an evaluation. Leroy et al. [3] encountered and documented this problem when evaluating machine learning algorithms. They compared three machine learning algorithms for word sense disambiguation in medical abstracts. A gold standard dataset provided by the National Library of Medicine (available at: http://wsd.nlm.nih.gov) was used. It focused on 50 ambiguous terms for which 100 instances were disambiguated by a team of 8 experts. It also contained a measure of agreement between experts for the disambiguation results. When the evaluation showed a ceiling effect, further investigation indicated that performance of the algorithms was related to the measure of agreement. More troublesome instances, i.e., instances with less agreement between experts, led to lower performance of the algorithms.

Finally, the use of a gold standard *may lead to over-fitting* when the standard was not general enough or when it was used for fine-tuning of the system. A gold standard created by one expert may reflect personal preferences. The gold standard may be very consistent, but evaluators should take into account that it reflects only one expert's opinion and so may reduce external validity. Once a gold standard is available, it is easy to evaluate many different versions of a system against it. Usually, once the first test has been conducted, the procedures for comparison will be easy to repeat and it becomes easy to test different versions of the system. For example, MS Excel macros may have been written to compare numeric output of an algorithm with a gold standard, or a database procedure may have been written to make the evaluation very efficient. The danger this holds is that a system will be developed and tuned that leads to extremely good performance for the given gold standard but it will lead to very poor performance with a new dataset.

It is important to keep in mind that few gold standards are perfect. Friedman [4] provides examples of different types of gold standards and evaluates their value using 'gold carats'. For example, when the outcome of a definitive test is used, a gold standard would receive a 23+ carat rating. On the other hand, a gold standard with substance abuse screening interviews gets only 10 carats. If the gold standard shows inconsistencies due to disagreement between experts, it does not mean the gold standard has become unusable. It may be less useful for machine learning applications but retain its value for other testing. When creating a gold standard with multiple experts, it is important to keep a record of any disagreements between them, their individual solutions and how a final decision was reached. When evaluating a system, it is acceptable to evaluate whether the system outcome agrees as much with the expert outcomes as the experts agree with each other.

Note that some developers may resort to machine-created gold standards because of the inconsistencies in the human-created versions. These standards are created by algorithms. Although this may result in better evaluation and results, researchers should take external validity into account and, ideally, follow up with an evaluation by humans. Machine-created gold standards may become unnaturally rigid and not representative of the natural, real environment. Algorithms may seem to perform exceptionally well because they only need to capture the systematic changes of the gold standard brought about by the standard-creating algorithms. When encountering real cases, subject to human error and variation, performance will be lower.

User Evaluation

Studies that do not rely on a gold standard require that the output of the algorithm or system is evaluated separately for each study. Studies involving user interactions are usually of this type. Although the outcome of a user study can also be compared against a gold standard, it is not commonly done. In this section, user evaluations are therefore contrasted with gold standard evaluations.

Frequently, user evaluations of an algorithm or information system do not rely on a gold standard but on people. Designing such user studies includes selecting the tasks to be done and the measurements for evaluation, recruiting the participants, conducting the study and, finally, evaluating and analyzing the results. Since one person can provide only one evaluation, it will be necessary to recruit several people to participate in the study. The type of design chosen will affect how many people are needed to complete the evaluation. With a between-subjects design (discussed in Chap. 4), each version of the system is tested by a different group of people. With a within-subjects design (discussed in Chap. 5), one group of people evaluates different versions of the system. Then, the researchers, developers or other external evaluators need to judge the output.

Who participates in the user evaluation can change depending on where in the system development life cycle the evaluation takes place. In the very early stages of development, the developers themselves may be the users. They will be able to judge whether the speed of the algorithms is sufficient, the results are reasonable and whether errors occur. However, it is clear that this may introduce bias because the evaluation leaves room for subjective judgments. Developers who have worked countless hours on the system may be providing a more positive judgment than could be expected from an objective observer. One should also keep potential conflicts of interest in mind, such as getting a bonus or being able to publish a paper based on good results. Or, a developer may have a more negative judgment than an objective observer would have. The developer may aim for perfection, which is often the start of feature creep in software development.

In many cases, a small dataset is used for the initial evaluations and it is reused until the system behaves as intended. Following this early testing, it is essential that new data is used for any follow-up evaluation regardless of who performs it, the developers or representative users. This is because system fitting to that particular dataset is likely to have occurred when data is used extensively. Continued use for formal testing would not be an honest evaluation of the system.

When the intended users cannot participate, developers should consider working with proxy users to conduct early testing. Although this is not optimal, when the proxy users are well chosen, they can still provide valuable feedback. For example, when developing a portable personal health record system for patients with HIV, several aspects of the system can be carried out with representative users who do not have HIV. Evaluating the ease of use of uploading scanned test results can be tested with adults belonging to the same demographic group as the population of HIV patients. The proxy users need to be representative of the intended users for as many characteristics as possible. For example, uploading files should not be measured with computer science students who would be much savvier at this task than the average adult.

Naturally, as the system development progresses, representative users need to be involved. Otherwise the evaluation will not possess external validity, and such systems will be in danger of failing when put in their intended environment.

Advantages

There are several advantages of conducting a user study in comparison to using a gold standard. Most important is that a user evaluation, when well designed and well conducted, provides a true estimate of how the information system would be used and what its impact would be. This cannot be easily deduced from gold standard evaluation, simulations or other types of studies.

A user evaluation can also be conducted at any point in the system development life cycle. The evaluation helps develop an information system that users want. Unwanted features can be identified and removed from the project; missing features can be added. It will also help developers learn what is important to users so they can devote their time accordingly.

Finally, a well designed user study will provide additional, high quality information above and beyond the measures taken. It often leads to ideas for future products, improvements in current products or design and sometimes even a first customer base.

Disadvantages

There are disadvantages to conducting user evaluations in comparison to using a gold standard. The first is that study participants need to be recruited. Furthermore, after designing the study, it may take additional resources to present the system in an environment that is suitably representative of the intended work environment and that allows collection of the evaluation data. For example, it may require adding tracking tools to the software to objectively record all user interactions with the system. A final disadvantage is a practical obstacle. When users are involved in an evaluation that will be published, most researchers will need to get approval from an Institutional Review Board. This may slow down the evaluation significantly.

Note that disadvantages of user studies are framed relative to gold standard evaluations and not presented in general. This is because although the studies cost time, money and effort, they lead to a high return on investment when they are well designed and executed by helping to create a much better product and preventing failure. This is so regardless whether it was developed in an academic or business environment.

References

1. Denny J, Peterson J, Choma N, Xu H, Miller R, Bastarache L, Peterson N (2010) Extracting timing and status descriptors for colonoscopy testing from electronic medical records. J Am Med Inform Assoc 17(4):383–388
2. Krallinger M, Morgan A, Smith L, Leitner F, Tanabe L, Wilbur J, Hirschman L, Valencia A (2008) Evaluation of text-mining systems for biology: overview of the second bio creative community challenge. Genome Biol 9(Suppl 2):S1. doi:doi:10.1186/gb-2008-9-s2-s1
3. Leroy G, Rindflesh TC (2005) Effects of information and machine learning algorithms on word sense disambiguation with small datasets. Int J Med Inform 74(7–8):573–585
4. Friedman CP, Wyatt JC (2000) Evaluation methods in medical informatics. Springer-Verlag, New York

Recruiting and Motivating Study Participants

10

Chapter Summary

This chapter provides tips on how to recruit and retain users for a study. When designing a user study, a lot of thought goes into choosing the variables, both dependent and independent, on top of the system design and development. An essential component that is sometimes overlooked until the last minute is the recruitment of participants for the study. Depending on where in the system's development life cycle the study takes place, the type of users, the number of users and the sampling strategies will change.

It is important that study participants are representative of the intended users of the system. The better they represent the intended system users, the more valuable their feedback will be. To accomplish this, it is discussed how to remove obstacles that would prevent people from participation, to be clear about expectations and to promote the contribution people make if it they participate. Money and other incentives used to motivate people to participate in the study are discussed, as well as the dangers this brings because such incentives may introduce bias. Finally, different sampling strategies that are possible and practical for studies in informatics are discussed. Random samples and stratified random samples are the gold standard, but convenience samples are often valuable for pilot studies and snowball sampling may be very helpful when more users are needed that fit a certain set of characteristics or when the study involves sensitive topics.

Type and Number of Participants

Recruitment is a time consuming activity. To avoid wasting time recruiting unsuitable participants, it is essential to consider the goals of the study being designed and how they relate to future studies. This is complicated in information system development since the development is cyclical. Multiple studies will be necessary. However, participants often cannot be invited to participate a second time in a study of the same system since it would lead to bias. Once people have participated, they may have formed an opinion about the system or may have been trained in a certain manner which would affect later studies.

Participant Characteristics

The researcher should think carefully about all future studies so that the most suitable users are invited for any particular study. Early in the development of an information system, basic characteristics that should apply to a broad group of people are usually evaluated and users without specific skills or characteristics can participate. When the system becomes increasingly fine-tuned for the intended user group, it will be essential to recruit representative users. Often, this becomes increasingly difficult, for example, with systems to be used by experts, ill people or people with very specific characteristics.

When designing the study, it is helpful to explicitly list the inclusion and exclusion criteria for participants. An explicit listing will help guide the recruitment process and facilitate ensuring a match between the goal of the study, the current status of the information system and the participants who will be recruited. For example, in pilot studies to evaluate communication software for children with autism spectrum disorder (ASD), the inclusion and exclusion criteria are extremely important since ASD is a spectrum disorder that has many different levels of severity. De Leo et al. [1] limited their studies to children with severe autism who were already introduced to a specific communication protocol, the Picture Exchange Communication System (PECS).

Researchers in the United States will have noticed that during the last decade federal agencies are requiring more inclusion of different user groups, for example, minorities and children, and explicit accounting for their inclusion.

Number of Participants

The number of participants required for a well designed study varies with the study goal. For an initial pilot study to verify the study design itself or to get initial reactions to the information system, a few participants may suffice. For example, a pilot study with 10 subjects can help capture many large problems if they exist. The number of subjects can also be small with usability studies. In the early 1990s, 4 or 5 was considered a large enough sample for such studies, although the number is creeping up with more complex websites and information systems being developed [2]. Others indicate that 8–12 evaluations of system-user interactions are usually sufficient to capture most (80%) of the problems [3]. Keep in mind that it will be difficult to discover all usability problems with a few users in one study.

To conduct a full-fledged experiment, enough subjects need to be recruited so that the experiment has enough power to show a significant difference between experimental conditions when it exists. A rule of thumb is that approximately 30 subjects are needed in each condition for this purpose. Note that this is not the number for the entire experiment. If there are three conditions, and the experiment uses a between-subjects design where each person participates in one experimental condition, then there will be about 30 people needed for each condition or 90 in total. For more precise numbers, the reader is referred to Chap. 2 where the power of experiments is discussed.

Since many subjects are needed for studies, delays in research are often due to slower-than-expected subject recruitment. For example, CenterWatch (www.center-watch.com), a Boston-based company, reviews clinical and research centers on a regular basis. It reports that slow patient enrollment is a major factor in delays in clinical trials.

Random Assignment

Randomization is important in user studies to ensure that bias and other unwanted effects are avoided or balanced out as much as possible. In practice, there are several ways to go about randomization. When deciding on the number of participants, it is best to include more people than strictly needed to counter the loss of participants due to attrition. Each participant is identified by means of an identification number, for example, 1 through N, and needs to be assigned to an experimental condition. Doing this before the start of the experiment allows the researcher to prepare all materials, programs and the environment in advance.

Modern methods to randomly assign participants to conditions mimic the earlier manual methods such as the roulette wheel method, flipping a coin or choosing a card from a shuffled deck. Random number generators make it possible to us a digital alternative to these methods. With the *roulette wheel method*, each experimental condition has an equal portion or slot on an imaginary roulette wheel. Probabilities can be used to simulate the roulette wheel. When the roulette wheel has a span 0–1, each experimental condition gets an equal portion of this span; with n conditions, there will be $1/n$ spans. Whenever a subject needs to be assigned, the wheel is spun by generation of a random number between 0 and 1. The slot on the wheel is selected that contains this number and the matching experimental condition is assigned to the subject.

For example, assume an independent variable "therapy" with 3 conditions: live therapist, computer therapist and self-help group. The roulette wheel has 3 slots, 1 for each condition, and each will be one-third of the total span. The live therapist condition is assigned the range 0–0.33, the computer therapist condition is assigned the range 0.34–0.66, and the self-help group condition is assigned the range 0.67–1. For each subject, the wheel is spun by generating a random number between 0 and 1. Depending on the number that is generated, a condition is assigned to the study subject. Thus, if the random probability assigned for the first subject is 0.78, this falls in the range of the third slot and the subject is assigned to the self-help group. If the random probability is 0.12, then the live therapist condition is assigned. The random numbers can be generated with a computer program, for example, MS Excel, or by consulting random number tables which are available in most statistical books [4–7].

In addition to mimicking the older methods, the subject participation numbers can also be assigned a random order directly. For example, if there are 120 subjects who will participate, the subject numbers s1, s2, ..., s120 can be randomly ordered. As a result, the order could be, for example, s13, s56, s1, ..., s82. The first group of 40 can then be assigned to the first condition, the second group to the second condition and the third group to the third condition. Or the condition could be randomly assigned to the first, second and third group. Once the random order has been decided for study participants, it can be used effectively to organize the study. Each participant is assigned a subject number (s1, s2, ...) and each subject number has been associated with an experimental condition.

Recruitment and Retention Tips

Recruitment and retention will be greatly improved if the researcher clearly defines the characteristics of the study sample and addresses potential obstacles to recruitment and retention. Items to consider are how to best reach potential participants and what would motivate them to participate. It is equally important to identify the obstacles faced by potential participants and to consider the additional obstacles particular to long term studies. Removing as many obstacles as possible will improve recruitment and retention. For successful recruitment it is essential to focus on the participants and how to facilitate their interaction instead of focusing on the researchers' convenience.

Advertise and Appeal

Use appropriate media to advertise. Depending on the intended subject sample, different media types will be more appropriate for subject recruitment. Some clinics or schools may have bulletin boards that people regularly read. Elderly people may be more prone to local or national printed media or periodicals. Younger groups rely more on the Internet and may be recruited there.

Explain the study in layman terms. When a study, its goals and procedures are explained in layman terms so that people can relate to it, it will be easier to recruit and retain participants. The explanation should include the study goal and how the participants will contribute to it, what the person's role will be and the time it will take. The language used to provide this information is very important. It needs to be understandable to laymen while still conveying enough information. With many studies, this is not easy. Unfortunately, there are no simple solutions to providing easy-to-understand explanations. Although the use of readability formulas is advocated to estimate the difficulty of text, their outcome has seldom been associated with actual understanding. Similar to providing medical information to patients or getting informed consent, the person's health literacy, the person's health status, the material used to provide information and the complexity of the topic, device or disease itself play a significant role.

Make both the appeal and the study relevant. When making the appeal to participate, the appeal itself should be interesting enough that the potential subjects read or listen to all that the researcher has to say. Using the best medium for the intended population will be an important factor in reaching people and increasing their interest in this. Making the study relevant is the next step. A personal interest in participating can be increased by using materials, tasks or systems that are characteristic and relevant to the potential subjects. Naturally, care should be taken that this does not lead to undue stress and concerns for the participants since that would lead to more dropouts. It may be wise to avoid sensitive topics. For example, when working with young adults on immersion games to increase physical exercise, the researchers should be careful not to overburden the participants with too much exercise. Similarly, when developing decision support tools for new mothers, the topics used during the study should be relevant but not unnecessarily alarming. Misinformation should be avoided as it will qualify as deception and complicate the study. At a minimum, additional protection of human subjects will need to be considered and approved by the Institutional Review Board (IRB).

Choose the best moment to invite people to participate. Timing is important. Make sure potential participants have time to listen, are not distracted and can concentrate on the invitation. For example, approaching patients who are waiting for their doctor's appointments is not a good strategy for immediate participation in a study, unless this is the group for which the system has been developed. These patients may be anxious, nervous, ill and stressed. Moreover, practical obstacles could keep them from participating. For example, they may be filling out paperwork prior to their doctor's appointment, making it impossible to interact with the researcher. They may also be called in for their appointment when the researcher is talking to them. If possible, it is better to wait until after their appointment to invite them to participate, regardless whether the request is for immediate participation or for setting a time for later.

Be Clear

Provide a clear description of the objectives of the study. When recruiting representative participants, the objective must be relevant and important to them. Explain the relevance of the research and the practical implications of the research in general and of their participation. Describe why they are a target population and why it is important that the study is conducted with representative people. Many people are very willing to help and advise when they are asked. By making it clear how they are helping the researcher, themselves and others like them, the researcher will have a much better chance of recruiting them.

Be clear about expectations. Potential participants should know what they are committing to and what they will get in return. Providing details about the duration of the study, frequency of interaction or intensity will help avoid attrition of study participants.

Remove Obstacles

Choose a time that is convenient for potential participants to participate in the study. Keeping all the advice in mind about making the participants and the environment as representative as possible, the chances of recruiting sufficient participants in a reasonable time frame will improve if the researcher schedules the study at a time that is convenient for the participants. For example, some patients may be coming into the hospital for dialysis. During the treatment, they may be bored and willing to spend their time helping someone else by participating in a study. Similarly, people who have just completed their doctor's visit will, most likely, be more willing than those who are waiting. Clinicians and researchers may be more inclined to give feedback if a study is organized during lunch and lunch is also provided.

Keep the study short. Don't make user studies overly long. When a study takes a very long time, participants will become tired and bored. In the worst case, they may stop giving the tasks or questions serious consideration and even start guessing. The maximum study duration depends on the participant characteristics and the type of study. Conducting a pilot study is crucial to ensure this boundary is not passed. A good starting point is 1 h as the maximum duration. Adjust this time for the study population, the task and the intensity of the study. Participants who are frail, very young, elderly or ill will require a shorter duration. If the tasks are considered boring, for example, filling out a long survey, some breaks should be included.

Facilitate transportation. Lack of, costly or inconvenient transportation is a serious obstacle for many people. Organizing or providing transportation or reimbursing the costs of transportation may make more subjects willing to participate. Alternatively, if the study can be conducted in situ, for example, at home or at a community center or retirement home, this major obstacle can be removed.

Facilitate making free time. Lack of free time due to work or elderly or childcare obligations is another major obstacle to participation. If the researcher is available to conduct studies after hours or provides childcare for the duration of the study, she will find many more people who are willing to participate. Conducting the study at a convenient time will also help with recruitment. For example, try conducting the study before or after work, therapy, clinic visits or gym sessions or around regular activities. Alternatively, getting permission to conduct a study at the work site or childcare center during appropriate hours may also help. Meals may also help with recruitment. Doing a study during lunch time and providing lunch may be an incentive by itself, and it may also help free up participants' time, since only the lunch period is used for the study.

Leverage Existing Resources

Recruit in local communities. It is helpful if the researcher can develop good relationships with existing communities. For example, retirement communities, libraries, community colleges, community centers, family clinics, community health centers [8], hospitals and even soup kitchens may be happy to participate. Miller et al. [9, 10] found that local staff at retirement homes and soup kitchens were often willing to facilitate advertising the study, for example, by posting the requests for participation, and even help with scheduling of the study, including reserving and providing a room.

Build a good relationship with communities. Local communities can be very valuable for multiple studies. Building a good relationship with them can be valuable both to the researcher and to the community. Building that relationship entails, minimally, that study results should be shared, explained and discussed. Keep the community abreast of any publications or results and acknowledge the participants in an appropriate manner. A little bit of extra effort often can help establish a better relationship that goes beyond one study. For example, the researchers may be in an excellent position to provide an unrelated service to these communities, such as serving as a (female) role model for high school students or volunteering time and effort in a soup kitchen. As usual, care should be taken that no bias is instituted in this manner. Naturally, not every researcher has the means to do this, and many other forms of interaction can show mutual respect and lead to good relationships.

Motivate

One of the practical problems seldom discussed in study design and statistical manuals is how to motivate the participants of the study. Imparting positive motivation during recruitment is key to recruiting enough participants for the study. Motivating subjects during the study is also important to avoid random or nonsense data. Unmotivated participants will negatively impact validity. Although payment is usually the first incentive that is considered when trying to motivate participants, other incentives exist that can be used.

Reimburse for time and effort. It is quite common to reimburse participants for their effort and time with money or with other incentives such as gift cards or tickets to events. Such payment should be used as a reimbursement for the time and effort spent to participate, but it should not be the sole motivating factor. Care should be taken that the compensation is appropriate for the group of participants so that this does not present undue influence and instigate bias. Offering too much money may influence people to participate when they otherwise would object. For example, if there are risks associated with participating, people could be coerced by money to participate. Payments may also lead to a biased sample of participants who partake in the study only for the money or because they need the money.

Give a prize or recognition for the best answer. In some cases, it is essential that participants do their best during the study. For example, when evaluating understanding of information, participants should be encouraged to give the best answers they can. Reimbursing for their time and requesting that they do their utmost may be insufficient motivation. In such cases, consider giving prizes for the best performance. Be aware that the motivation will be different for different groups of participants. For example, a $15 prize will not be very motivating for a medical doctor who may prefer another type of recognition. On the other hand, it may be very effective with participants in soup kitchens or homeless shelters.

The extra incentives require additional organization because they can only be given after completion of the study, and confidentiality of personal information should remain guaranteed. There exist several options however. One option is to provide participants with a unique identifying number that appears on their study materials. They do not have to give any extra information but only need to take their number with them. The best scores with the unique numbers can be posted on a website or communicated in another manner, such as mail, a notice on a bulletin board or email, to all participants so that those with the matching numbers can collect their prize. Alternatively, participants can write a code name on their study materials which only they will remember. The information about the best scores can be conveyed in the same manner. Alternatively, a separate sheet can be retained that combines the code names or numbers with actual contact information. This last option makes it possible for the researcher to contact the persons or send them their prize. This may be the preferred option if no bulletin boards or Internet sites can be used, when a large group of participants would be calling in or stopping by to check on their results or when it is preferred that the researcher initiates the contact.

Payments will influence the participants. There are documented cases where participants fabricated information to be able to participate in a study they considered to pay well or where they refused to partake because they believed the amount of money they could earn was insufficient [11]. Ripley [11] reviewed several studies for the impact of participation payments. Focusing on questionnaire-based substance abuse, HIV risk reduction and hypertension studies, she demonstrated the possibility of both positive and negative consequences but also potential sources for bias in the data as a result of payments or lack of payments. She also showed how the impact differs depending on personal characteristics of the participants, such as age, income and health status. As can be expected, healthy subjects react differently to study benefits than ill people. The healthy participants were more influenced by the payment. Different age groups also act differently depending on the payment offered, with younger people being more motivated by the payment. Note that these results are all based on self-reported motivation and what participants volunteered as their reasons for participating.

Researchers should ask participants whether they are concurrently participating in other studies or have previously participated in studies. Although they need to rely on the honesty of the participants, the question is worth asking. Dishonest participants will not easily be caught. But knowledge of the subjects' participation in multiple studies, even when acceptable for the current study, can help interpret results. These people may exhibit a different profile or may experience unexpected interaction effects, especially in the realm of medical devices or therapy. In the evaluation of information systems, the negative effect of participating in multiple information system evaluations will be in having potential bias for or against a system.

With longitudinal studies send regular updates on the progress of the study. These updates can take many forms: a letter, personal visits or a phone call. In addition to the updates, information and reminders can be included about future or continuing participation.

Provide other benefits such as medications, tests or medical exams. When other benefits are provided to study participants, they may be a motivating factor even if it is not the main intention to use them as such. For example, for some patients, participating in studies may be the only way to get a new test or medication. The same caution should be used with these benefits as with monetary incentives.

Sampling Methods

When conducting studies in informatics, the sample and population that are relevant to the study can be comprised of people or artifacts. Messages written by people, health records, diagnostic test results and images are artifacts. In most studies, it will be impossible to evaluate all existing people or artifacts and so a subset is selected: the sample. A variety of sampling methods is discussed below. Since different sampling methods have been shown to lead to different characteristics being more or less present in the sample, a good list of descriptive statistics, such as age, occupation, race and educational level, is essential to evaluate any user study. For example, Schwarcz et al. [12] compared two sampling methods systematically when evaluating the sexual behaviors, substance abuse and HIV testing behaviors of men who have sex with men using a survey approach. They compared a probabilistic sample and a convenience sample. Among their findings was that substance abuse was higher in the convenience sample. However, they found that the two groups displayed differences in their demographic characteristics. The men in the probability sample were older, better educated and had higher incomes than those in the convenience sample.

Not all possible methods are included in this section because many of the existing sampling plans are suitable for survey-based research but very difficult for user studies involving the evaluation of information systems. In survey-based research, the entire population is often known. In this case, a random sample from the population can be invited to participate. This is not so with the evaluation of information systems where a typical user is envisioned. The entire population is not known, not reachable or not accessible. Similarly, in survey-based research it is sometimes possible to estimate the characteristics of participants in a population. The characteristics of the sample can then be compared against these and conclusions can be adjusted as necessary. Finding such differences has also led to the explicit comparison of different sampling plans, such as time-location sampling and respondent-driven sampling, for their effects on participant characteristics [13]. There are also practical obstacles that make the sampling different. For example, installing an information system in a randomly selected hospital will be impossible.

As in all fields, in informatics it is important to keep in mind that the sample of people or their artifacts should be representative of the entire population. How the sample is selected will affect the validity of the results. When the sample is not representative or is biased, the conclusions cannot be generalized to the intended populations. Sampling methods are therefore an important aspect to consider when designing a user study.

Random Sampling

In informatics, the term *random sampling* is frequently used when a sample is taken from a large set of people or artifacts but not necessarily sampled from the entire population. In many cases, the entire population is not available to be contacted but a sufficiently large subpopulation is available and can be reached. A random sample is a subset of units taken in such a manner that each unit has an equal chance of being selected. The units also need to be selected independently from each other. Today, this can be done very practically by assigning numbers to units and using a random number generator to select the numbers. For example, using the phone book or some registry, a large group of people may be selected in a random fashion. Gong and Zhang [14] used such an approach to randomly select participants for the user interface study of their Hyperlipidemia Management System. The invited people were randomly selected via the internal email system at the University of Texas Health Science Center at Houston.

With electronic storage of requests, responses, information and records of many types, there is much opportunity to conduct experiments that include random samples of data. For example, Solberg et al. [15] evaluate the effects of a decision support system (DSS) on requests for high-tech diagnostic imaging procedures. Their independent variable was the information technology which had two levels: no DSS and the EHR DSS. They measured the level of appropriateness of the requests, abnormal findings and apparent effects on patient care. The sample was randomly selected from the orders that were placed before or after the implementation of the EHR decision support system. There was no effect on the proportion of positive findings or on patient impact, but they did find that tests ordered after implementation fit the appropriateness requirements.

Stratified Random Sampling

Stratified random sampling is a technique used when a population contains different subgroups, called clusters or strata, which may react differently to the independent variable. To get a representative sample of such a population, it is essential that there are representatives of each group in the sample. To ensure this, a stratified random sample can be drawn. To use such a sampling technique, the group is divided into subgroups and a random sample is then taken from each subgroup. One or more variables can be used to define the groups. For example, Bergman et al. [16] stratified their sample by age for each gender and randomly selected and then invited 200 men and 200 women from the predefined age groups to participate in the study. The study used and compared survey-based measures of alcohol use and computer-tomographic-based measures of cerebral disorder.

When the proportions of each group in the total population are known, then these proportions may also be represented in the stratified sample so that the same proportions are found in the sample as in the population. The resulting sample is called a *weighted stratified random sample*. With many surveys being conducted and datasets available, there are many studies that apply this strategy to select their sample. For example, Lam and Lam [17] evaluate the Internet usage among older caregivers in Australia using a stratified random sample taken from the responses to a national survey.

Convenience Sampling

Convenience sampling, also called *accidental sampling*, relies on a method that is not explicitly designed to recruit participants representative of the population but instead takes advantage of location, circumstances or other opportunities which may present themselves. The sample is recruited in a manner that was convenient for the researcher at the time.

The main advantage of this approach is the convenience. However, convenience samples are prone to different types of bias. If the convenience was due to a specific location or event, such as a free health screening, the study conclusions have to be moderated and are only valid for the population represented by the sample. Depending on the study purpose, the effect of bias may be more or less pronounced. For example, when evaluating whether encouraging text messages are seen as positive with a group of gym goers, there may be a systematic higher rating because they already are actively involved in managing their health as is shown by their gym attendance. In contrast, if the study is about understanding health literature, then demographic questions can verify whether the sample is representative of the national population.

As always, the researcher needs to decide what the best sampling method is and to compare the advantages with other potential methods. In some cases, there is little difference between the techniques. For example, when a student asks persons in the same classroom to participate, this is a convenience sample. If the intended population consists of students, this convenience sample may result in a fair representation of the population. However, because of the many potential biases, this type of sampling is considered more useful for pilot studies than for full-blown studies.

Snowball Sampling

Snowball sampling relies on referrals. This type of sampling is useful when more participants of a particular group are needed. Participants who have agreed to take part in a study may refer others to the study or they may provide contact information of people in their network to be approached for participation. For example, snowball sampling was used to survey public facilities and their computer access in an effort to understand factors that contribute to a digital divide between the general population and those with cognitive disabilities [18]. Recently, snowball sampling is being used in online social networks by making use of existing links between people.

An advantage of this approach is that it may be easier to recruit people when they are introduced to the study by someone they value or trust. For example, Luk et al.[19] used snowball sampling starting with only a few rural and urban doctors for their telemedicine studies in Ghana. Since they studied knowledge sharing among professionals, such trust was essential in being able to recruit enough participants. Snowball sampling may also be more effective with sensitive topics. For example, Sheu et al. [20] conducted a study on medication administration errors. They used snowball sampling techniques to recruit a sufficient number of nurses. Snowball sampling can also be a practical approach when there exists a champion who is committed to getting the study done. For example, if the champion is a department head, teacher, team leader or otherwise responsible for different people who qualify for participation in the study, this champion can make it easier for them to participate, for example, by allowing time for the study during normal work hours.

Naturally, the disadvantage of this approach is that a lot of the recruitment process is not controlled by the researchers. For example, since it is not the researcher who extends the study invitations, it is unknown how many people did not participate, making it harder to judge a potential selection bias. It is also difficult to control which message is used to invite people to participate. This message may set expectations about the study and what will be evaluated. Moreover, the number of people who will be recruited will depend on the skills and connections of those used to start the sample. And depending on who is inviting, for example, supervisors inviting employees, the sample may be more or less representative and not always voluntary.

Sampling Bias

When people make up the sampling units, it is very difficult to get an unbiased sample. It is easier to get a random sample when the sampling units are, for example, electronic health records, diagnostic tests or websites. In such cases, once the entire collection has been made available, selecting a random sample is trivial. When a sample is not completely random, that is, when not all units have equal opportunity to be selected and participate in the study, the sample is biased. Understanding the potential bias is essential when drawing conclusions about the population based on the sample.

An important reason why many user studies often suffer from a selection bias is that the researcher has to rely on volunteers to participate in the research. As can be expected, not every person is willing to participate in a study. If the sample of volunteers is not representative of the population, the validity of the conclusions will be in doubt. Volunteers self-select to participate and this group may share characteristics that are different from non-volunteers. This may be especially pronounced in studies that measure opinions. It may be only the people with an opinion, sometimes only those with a strong opinion, who volunteer. With other studies where behaviors or achievements are measured, people who expect to score differently from others may prefer not to participate. For example, when a person is not computer-savvy, he will be less likely to participate voluntarily in a study using computers.

The differences between volunteers and non-volunteers have been the topic of several psychology studies. An important conclusion that can be drawn from the research on volunteers and non-volunteers in research is that differences exist. Rosenthal and Rosnow [5] list 17 characteristics that have been found to differ between the two groups. Some examples are that volunteers tend to be better educated than non-volunteers, have higher social class status, higher need for social approval, are more sociable and less authoritarian. Depending on the type of research, there are other characteristics that differ. For example, for general research, the volunteers tend to be more intelligent, but for non-typical research, such as research on hypnosis or personality research, this is not the case. It is essential to be aware of these existing biases.

Recruiting and motivating participants is an important activity in a user study. Without them, the study cannot take place. However, care is needed to ensure that those who do participate and complete the study are sufficiently representative to allow valid conclusions and generalizations.

References

1. De Leo G, Gonzales C, Battagiri P, Leroy G (2010) A smart-phone application and a companion website for the improvement of the communication skills of children with autism: clinical rationale, technical development and preliminary results. J Med Syst 1:1–9
2. Bastien JMC (2010) Usability testing: a review of some methodological and technical aspects of the method. Int J Med Inform 79:e18–e23
3. Kushniruka AW, Patel VL (2004) Cognitive and usability engineering methods for the evaluation of clinical information systems. J Biomed Inform 37:56–76
4. Vaughan L (2001) Statistical methods for the information professional: a practical, painless approach to understanding, using, and interpreting statistics. commercial statistics. Information Today, Inc, New Jersey
5. Rosenthal R, Rosnow RL (1991) Essentials of behavioral research: Methods and data analysis. McGraw-Hill, Boston
6. Kirk RE (1995) Experimental design: procedures for the behavioral sciences, 3rd edn. Brooks/Cole Publishing Company, Pacific Grove
7. Kurtz NR (1999) Statistical analysis for the social sciences. Social sciences - statistical methods. Allyn & Bacon, Needham Heights
8. Glynn SM, Randolph E, Garrick T, Lui A (2010) A proof of concept trial of an online psychoeducational program for relatives of both veterans and civilians living with schizophrenia. Psychiatr Rehabil J 33(4):278–287
9. Miller T (2008) Dynamic generation of a health topics overview from consumer health information documents and its effect on user understanding, memory, and recall. Doctoral dissertation, Claremont Graduate University, Claremont
10. Miller T, Leroy G (2008) Dynamic generation of a health topics overview from consumer health information documents. Int J Biomed Eng Technol 1(4):395–414
11. Ripley EBD (2006) Journal of Empirical Research on Human Research Ethics: An International Journal 1(4):9–20

12. Schwarcz S, Spindler H, Scheer S, Valleroy L, Lansky A (2007) Assessing representativeness of sampling methods for reaching men who have sex with men: a direct comparison of results obtained from convenience and probability samples. AIDS Behav 11:596–602. doi:10.1007/s10461-007-9232-9

13. Kendall C, Kerr LRFS, Gondim RC, Werneck GL, Macena RHM, Pontes MK, Johnsto LG, Sabin K, McFarland W (2008) An empirical comparison of respondent-driven sampling, time location sampling, and snowball sampling for behavioral surveillance in men who have sex with men, Fortaleza, Brazil. AIDS Behav 12:S97–S104. doi:doi:10.1007/s10461-008-9390-4

14. Gong Y, Zhang J (2009) Toward a human-centered hyperlipidemia management system: the interaction between internal and external information on relational data search. J Med Syst. doi:10.1007/s10916-009-9354-x

15. Solberg LI, Wei F, Butler JC, Palattao KJ, Vinz CA, Marshall MA (2010) Effects of electronic decision support on high-tech diagnostic imaging orders and patients. Am J Manag Care 16(2):102–106

16. Bergman H, Axelsson G, Ideström C-M, Borg S, Hindmarsh T, Makower J, Mützell S (1983) Alcohol consumption, neuropsychological status and computer-tomographic findings in a random sample of men and women from the general population. Pharmacol Biochem Behav 18(Supplement 1):501–505

17. Lam L, Lam M (2009) The use of information technology and mental health among older caregivers in Australia. Aging Ment Health 13(4):557–562

18. Fox LE, Sohlberg MM, Fickas S, Lemoncello R, Prideaux J (2009) Public computing options for individuals with cognitive impairments: survey outcomes. Disabil Rehabil Assist Technolnology 4(5):311–320

19. Luk R, Ho M, Aoki PM (2008) Asynchronous remote medical consultation for Ghana. In: Proceeding of the twenty-sixth annual SIGCHI conference on human factors in computing systems, Florence, Italy, 2008. ACM, pp 743–752

20. Sheu S, Wei I, Chen C, Yu S, Tang F (2009) Using snowball sampling method with nurses to understand medication administration errors. J Clin Nurs 18(4):559–569

Institutional Review Board (IRB) Approval

11

Chapter Summary

The Institutional Review Board (IRB) has to approve most studies that involve human subjects. This chapter first discusses the origin of the Institutional Review Board, which goes back as far as World War II when experiments were conducted on prisoners, to illustrate how different historical events resulted in an official review being required for experimentation on human subjects. Then, the components of the information submitted for review are discussed. This includes the study rationale, its design and how data are to be gathered and published. In addition, special attention is paid to the need for the study participants to provide informed consent. For participants to be able to give such consent the researcher needs to provide all necessary information, participants need to be able understand it and then need to agree to taking part in the study. This process is not without its consequences and has been shown to affect the timeliness of research, the study's recruitment success and also the representativeness of the study sample.

Origin of the IRB

The Institutional Review Board is a team of the researcher's peers that oversees the aspects of ongoing research that involve human subjects. The concept of such a review board came into existence, along with many other ethics boards, in response to several separate historical events. Although these boards have existed for decades, today there is still a current and ongoing discussion of their involvement with and effects on ongoing research.

The main event leading to the creation of the IRB was the Nuremberg trial of Nazi doctors. This trial had an impact across the world, and the resulting principles have been adopted in several national and international ethics codes and guidelines. During World War II, several doctors working in German prison camps used prisoners as test subjects. Experiments were conducted on the prisoners without their consent, under inhuman circumstances which often resulted in prisoners dying or

G. Leroy, *Designing User Studies in Informatics*, Health Informatics,
DOI 10.1007/978-0-85729-622-1_11, © Springer-Verlag London Limited 2011

being maimed for life. After the war, in 1945, the International Military Tribunal was held in Nuremberg, Germany. The initial trial was held for the Nazi leadership, but it was then followed by additional trials of 23 Nazi doctors. At its completion in 1947, 15 were found guilty and several were sentenced to death.

The Nuremberg trial is relevant to today's IRB because of the *Nuremberg Code* that was one of the outcomes of this trial. The Nuremberg code was the ethical standard against which the defendants had been measured and it still forms the basis of reviews of experimentation with humans today. The reference to the full code can be found in the next chapter (Chap. 12). Its principles are summarized below:

1. Voluntary consent of the subject participant.
2. The study should lead to results for the good of the society.
3. The study should take previous knowledge into account so that executing the study is justified.
4. The study should avoid unnecessary physical and mental suffering or injury.
5. The study should not be conducted when there is a reason to believe that death or disabling injury may occur as a result of the study. A possible exception is where the researcher is the subject.
6. The risk involved with the study should not exceed that determined by the humanitarian importance of the problem and the contribution to its solution by the experiment.
7. The study should be conducted so that participants are protected from even remote possibilities of injury, disability or death.
8. A qualified person should conduct the study.
9. A subject should be able to quit the study at any time when the subject decides further participation is no longer possible for physical or mental reasons.
10. The researcher should be prepared to and should in effect end the study at any stage if continuation may lead to injury, disability or death of the subject.

A second important cornerstone that led to formal protection of human subjects in experiments is the *Declaration of Helsinki*. The Declaration of Helsinki has been adopted in many countries across the world as the ethical standard for physicians. It originates with the World Medical Association, which is comprised of national medical associations and represents millions of physicians worldwide. It contains the principles from the Nuremberg Code and several clarifications. The first version was adopted in 1964 and has been revised several times.

In addition to the World Medical Association, the *Council for International Organizations of Medical Sciences* (CIOMS) also created ethical guidelines. This council is an international nonprofit, nongovernmental organization that was established in 1949 by the World Health Organization (WHO) and the United Nations Educational, Scientific and Cultural Organization (UNESCO). In 1993 the council published its International Ethical Guidelines for Biomedical Research Involving Human Subjects, which was subsequently revised and updated in 2002.

In addition to the events during World War II and the resulting ethical guidelines by international organizations, there were additional events which helped shape the institutional review process. Two well known events are the Thalidomide tragedy and the Tuskegee Syphilis study [1]. The *Thalidomide tragedy* involved the use of a sedative, Thalidomide, which was not approved by the U.S. Food and Drug Administration (FDA) at the time of the study but was handed out as samples to physicians. Physicians subsequently prescribed it to their patients including pregnant women. Many people taking the drug were not aware it was not approved by the FDA and that it was an experimental substance. Nobody had consented to participating in such an experiment. It turned out that the drug was extremely harmful to fetal development, which resulted in birth defects, especially when taken during the first trimester of pregnancy.

The second such impactful event was the *Tuskegee Syphilis study* which was conducted over many years starting in 1932. The goal of this study was to learn the consequences of not treating syphilis. At the time, the treatment was sometimes more devastating than the disease. A county and hospital which showed high rates of syphilis were selected and black male subjects were invited to participate. They were told they had 'bad blood', which was a local expression at the time to cover a variety of diseases. The study went on for several years during which study subjects did not receive any treatment. They were even exempted from military service so that the measurement of the effects of untreated syphilis could be continued. Meanwhile, penicillin was discovered as an accepted cure for syphilis. Shockingly, the subjects, who had not even been told about their disease, were also withheld treatment.

Both studies resulted in physically damaging effects, but other studies that focused on mental processes also played a role in the creation of institutional reviews for experimentation on humans. The most famous example is the series of *Milgram studies* [2, 3]. These experiments were conducted to evaluate obedience in humans. Study participants 'played' the role of teacher and had to administer shocks to other participants who needed to memorize words. Unknown to the participant, this learner was an actor who did not receive any shocks but pretended to be incorrect and hurt by the shocks. Not only was it appalling how far participants were willing to go in the experiment, many delivered the maximum shock while the learner appeared to be unconscious and then explained their behavior as correct because they were 'just following instructions'. This type of behavior was found in a variety of situations, ranging from environments such as university laboratories to much shadier environments with doubtful researchers.

In 1974, when the U.S. Congress passed the *National Research Act*, the National Commission for the Protection of Human Subjects of Biomedical and Behavioral Research was created. This commission wrote the *Belmont Report*, a set of principles for regulating protection of human rights. The report is not intended as a set of rules but as a standard that recognizes that the decision process in medical research is not always easy or clear cut. The report specifies three principles: *respect for persons* (also referred to as *autonomy*), *beneficence* and *justice*. Adhering to the first principle, respect for the person, means that each person participating in research should be treated as an individual with autonomy. When that person's autonomy is diminished, for example, in the case of children or prisoners, the person is entitled to protection. This principle also specifies that the person needs to give informed consent before participating in the study, indicating that he or she understands what will or will not happen by participating. The second principle, beneficence, stipulates that researchers are obliged to protect the participants from harm and that the benefits of participating should be maximized while possible harms should be minimized. The third principle, justice, refers to fairness. Inclusion and exclusion criteria should be fair, and diverse populations should be included in the study. This third rule does not preclude randomization of subjects to conditions. However, the randomization process will need to be explained during informed consent.

In addition to international and national standards, several professional organizations have their own ethics code. These codes commonly reflect principles similar to those of the Nuremberg Code and the Declaration of Helsinki. Several academic journals and research institutions apply their own additional rules to ensure the protection of human subjects during experimentation.

Who Needs Permission

Most academic institutions across the world require review of studies involving human subjects to verify they comply with ethical guidelines. All researchers who receive funding from the U.S. Department of Health and Human Services (DHHS) are required to submit their research studies to their IRB for review when they involve human subjects. In addition, most research institutions in the United States require their researchers to comply with federal rules for all studies that involve human subjects, regardless of the funding sources, and submit to IRB review. Besides academic institutions, there are also several professional organizations, for example the American Psychological Association (APA), that have developed rules and standards for ethical conduct that their members need to adhere to when conducting research that involves human subjects. Finally, some academic journals also require review of research with human subjects by an IRB if the researchers are considering publishing their results in the journal. For example, the *IEEE Transactions on Biomedical Circuits and Systems* requires documentation that the research on human subjects was conducted in accordance with the Helsinki Declaration.

There are different levels of review that can be conducted by an IRB. Although all guidelines should be followed by the researcher, in some cases the potential for harm is very small and such a study may be excluded from full board review. The research study may qualify for an expedited review, which means that only one member and not the complete board reviews the application. Research projects can qualify for expedited review if the research poses minimal risk, is not classified research, does not lead to identification of subjects with potential harm as a result and if the research belongs to one of nine categories. For the exact details, the reader should check the guidelines provided by the Department of Health and Human Services and her own research institution. The references to this information are provided in the next chapter (Chap. 12). An overview of the nine categories of research which may be exempt from full review follows. Note that this list is not limited to studies in informatics but includes all categories:

1. Clinical studies that involve drugs for which an investigational new drug application is not required, studies that involve medical devices for which an investigational device exemption application is not required or a medical device that has been approved for marketing and which is used in accordance with that approval.

2. Studies that use collections of blood samples collected by finger, heel or ear stick or venipuncture from healthy, non-pregnant adults with a weight of at least 110 lb. A smaller amount can be used from other human subjects, keeping restrictions in mind such as the age and health of the subject.

3. Studies that collect biological specimens, for example, hair and nail clippings, for research using noninvasive means.

4. Studies using data collected through noninvasive procedures routinely used in medical practice, with the exception of x-rays or microwaves. For example, by using physical sensors on the body, testing senses, electrocardiography and electroencephalography, among others.

5. Studies using data, records or specimens that are collected for purposes other than research.

6. Studies with data collected from recording done for research purposes using voice, video or images.

7. Studies on characteristics or behaviors, or studies using surveys or interviews conducted in groups or individually.

8. Studies that have been approved already and continue beyond the original timeline and where either no new subjects are recruited, the research activities are complete or there is long-term follow-up of subjects, or where no subjects were enrolled but no additional risk is identified, or where only data analysis remains to be done.

9. Studies with minimal risk, even if they do not belong in the above categories, that have been reviewed by the IRB and labeled as having minimal risk.

There are also studies that may be exempt from any review by the IRB. However, even for research that is exempt, an institution may require notification of the projects and a short description. The reader is referred to the next chapter (Chap. 12) for references to the Code of Federal Regulations of the Department of Health and Human Services. In short, the following research may be exempt:

1. Research in normal educational settings. For example, when evaluating a new teaching method of which the results will not be submitted for publication but only reviewed in-house.

2. Research using educational tests, surveys or interviews and research based on observing public behavior if the human subjects cannot be individually identified.

3. Research on secondary use of de-identified, existing datasets. For example, data mining on existing datasets or use of existing datasets as gold standards for evaluation when this is available without identification information.

4. Evaluations that are not considered 'research', such as in-house program evaluations or evaluations of public benefit and service programs.

5. Taste and food quality evaluation (for 'normal' food).

6. Research that does not involve human subjects. For example, comparing the outcome of algorithms for errors, speed, etc.

Many researchers in informatics believe their research is exempt from review. This is the case when evaluating websites and communication from public online communities that are not password protected and no individually identifiable data will be reported. The information can be considered to be public behavior and is visible to everyone. Although this type of research may be exempt, the researcher should keep the principles in mind and not unduly expose individuals. Caution should be used with publicly posted video, chats and images [4]. For example, when using images from Internet sites, care should be taken to protect the identity of the creators. IRB review may be necessary to ensure confidentiality is guaranteed, even if the data is anonymized for the research. Other types of information, such as network data, photos with tags and serial numbers or webpage edit trails, for example, for Wikipedia, that may lead to personal identification may also pose problems.

IRB and Other Review Boards

Researchers in informatics are seldom trained or informed about the need for IRB review. However with interdisciplinary research becoming increasingly the norm, it is essential for researchers and developers to understand the workings of the IRB and what its role is. In addition, with more informatics experiments involving human participants, IRB review becomes part of this process, all the more since information systems are increasingly used in medicine, psychology and education where privacy and safety are of the utmost concern.

In the U.S., the IRB overseeing academic research is usually located at a university. However, there also exist several independent review boards; a list of them is included in the next chapter (Chap. 12). Some of these boards are for-profit organizations, usually without governmental oversight, and some are paid by pharmaceutical companies whose independence is questionable to some researchers. In other countries, the rules are not always as explicitly defined as in the U.S. and not always interpreted as broadly. However, most accept the Nuremberg Code and the Declaration of Helsinki as standards and have associated laws to regulate experimentation with human subjects. Comparable to the U.S., those research institutions have their own local rules and regulations. In addition, the rules may be established and enforced by an ethics commission. And experiments in the behavioral sciences, such as psychology, usually must adhere to the local interpretations of their professional associations' ethical rules.

The IRB should be independent of the researchers submitting the application, the sponsors of the research and also of any monetary, material or other benefit related to the research. Although seldom mentioned, it would be ideal if the IRB members were also from a different institution or university because, as Macklin [5] points out, independence is broader than the material benefits but should also include social constraints. The members on the board have significant power to delay or stop a research study. This may be tempting when the board members are evaluating competing research. Another reason is that while IRB oversight of research helps protect human rights in research, IRB review and continued involvement may help discover and stop fraud or other types of misconduct [6].

Discussions are ongoing about the need to change the makeup of the boards in response to the use of evaluation in informatics studies. There is a need for at least some board members to have a basic understanding of computing [7]. There is also a plea to make the response time faster so that IRB review is more in tune with the fast pace in informatics [4]. For example, when testing algorithms that can detect deception and lying, humans may be asked to play the role of hackers. They play against the computer. Similarly, study participants can be asked to lie to test an automated interview system. The IRB needs to understand that the algorithms or information systems are being tested using artifacts, for example, fabricated lies. Even with this type of artifact-based evaluation of information system components, different levels of review may be prescribed, ranging from being exempt or an expedited review to a full review. It is the researcher's responsibility to verify which approval is necessary at the institution where the experiment will be conducted, and it is the board's responsibility to have a basic understanding of such research so that reasonable review can be conducted.

Two types of research may require additional review over and above the IRB review discussed in this chapter. Although not discussed in detail in this section, they are mentioned to complete the list. The first is genetic research for which there are additional, specific guidelines provided by the National Institutes of Health (NIH) and the Institutional Biosafety Committee (IBC) that oversees this work. Although private institutions are not bound by these rules, most will follow them to ensure enhanced protection of human subjects. The second type is clinical trials which may require additional oversight. This oversight is provided by a Data Monitoring Committee (DMC). The two committees mentioned here came into existence in the 1960s to provide in-process monitoring. They were originally referred to as Data Safety Monitoring Boards (DSMB) and are necessary where mortality or morbidity are the primary or secondary endpoints [1].

IRB Components for Information Systems Evaluation

Acquiring IRB approval may be daunting, but understanding the principles behind it makes the process manageable and faster. The first task the researcher should do is become familiar with the institution, company or funder's requirements for IRB review including the procedures, forms and timelines. In some cases, the studies will be reviewed by the medical IRB, while in other cases the behavioral sciences IRB will review the study. Most research institutions today will have their procedures online. When IRB review is required, it needs to be completed and the study approved before the study can start. The details of how the Institutional Review Board (IRB) conducts its business are different at every institution, but application forms together with submission deadlines are usually all available to researchers online.

The application process typically consists of a set of forms that need to be completed, dated and signed by the researcher. The forms contain questions about the purpose of the study, experimental design, how consent will be gained and how participants and their experimental data will be protected. Protection of participants includes both physical protection and protecting participants from misuse of their data. This is usually accomplished by making the data confidential. *Confidentiality* means that private information is not shared in public and not used for purposes other than the originally stated purpose. In research, data can be kept confidential if only aggregates of the data are shown in such a manner that no single individual can be identified. Note the difference with privacy, which is the right to keep information about oneself to oneself, in other words, the right not to share that information. While in many places the forms will be a list of structured questions and fill-in-the-blanks sections, other institutions allow free text submissions. The required information often includes, but is not necessarily limited to:

- Background and objectives of the study.
- Study design including an explanation of independent and dependent variables.
- Study population and sample including the inclusion and exclusion criteria.
- Recruitment methods, including approval to recruit if this is done at a non-public location.
- Data analysis methods.
- Benefits, risk and risk management approach.
- Records and information kept including information about how information is to be stored and kept confidential.
- Informed consent letter or other materials and the process followed.

Once the information has been completed and submitted, the IRB reviews the proposed study, accepts or rejects the application or requires clarifications and modifications. The timeliness of review, the amount of details requested and the duration of the entire process depends on the institution. Especially with medical research, IRBs instigate strict rules to protect patient privacy and safety. Some universities may also have other institutions conduct their IRB review. For example, the U.S. National Institutes of Health's National Cancer Institute (NCI) supports local IRBs in the review process with its Centralized IRB Initiative. This service is intended to help research institutions speed up the research process.

With the exception of the informed consent form, the information required for the IRB review is largely the same as that to design the study and can be found in this book. However, gaining informed consent requires additional attention. Most studies in informatics are straightforward. Even so, the principles of human research need to be followed. The principles discussed above are the cornerstone of review and impact the informed consent process. The first principle was the principle of respect for the person, which requires researchers to provide information at the start of the study so that potential subjects can make an informed decision about participating or withdrawing from the study. Because such informed consent is difficult to accomplish in medicine and computing, where many of the concepts are difficult to understand for potential subjects, special attention should be paid to this process.

Informed Consent Information

There are three important steps in the informed consent process. The first step is that the potential subject receives sufficient information about the study. This means that the person has to understand the project is research and not an established treatment or therapy. Any potential risks, harm or discomfort that can be expected from participating must be explained. Furthermore, the study itself has to be described together with its purpose. This includes meta-information about the study, such as the expected duration of the study and the subject's participation. It also includes information about how and why the study may be terminated by the researchers, or how and why a participant can terminate the study, together with potential consequences of termination. For example, in an educational setting there should be no consequences to course grades or chances of graduating if a subject needs to terminate participation in a study. However, in a study where medical devices are used or medication is given, terminating participation may have consequences that need to be explained. The consent material should also explain how data will be treated, how it will be stored and shared, and who will have access to it. It is often important to potential subjects to know how many subjects are to be recruited. For example, for research on rare diseases with very few known sufferers, participation in the study may be vital. People appreciate this type of information and may be more inclined to continue participation when they realize how valuable their participation is. Moreover, in studies where thousands of participants are recruited, the summary statistics are based on many people which may be a factor of comfort. Finally, it is also important to provide contact information so that potential subjects can ask questions about the study before, during and after participation. It is good practice to inform participants at this point in the process about how they may learn of the results at the end of the study.

The second step to be completed for a valid informed consent process is to ensure the ability of the participant to understand the given information. This is probably the most difficult part of the process, especially with complex studies or studies that involve deception. The study information is commonly distributed by means of text. Several examples can be seen for clinical trials at ClinicalTrials.gov. Providing a description in layman's language is difficult but necessary. Therefore, the researcher should not limit this process to the use of text but can add other means, such as in-person explanation or video and images, to facilitate understanding. An important part of this step is to give the person enough time to digest the information and make a decision. Especially with studies running over a long period of time, consent may need to be split in different sections and asked anew when the study proceeds to a new phase.

Finally, the third step that is necessary in an informed consent process is that the potential subject gives his or her consent voluntarily. The informed consent process should be executed by a person with the necessary authority to sign up participants and sufficient knowledge about the study to answer questions correctly. This does not mean that the researcher should be this person. In some cases, another person is the better choice to avoid undue influence. For example, when there is a pre-existing or continuing relationship between researcher and participant or when the potential subject is a subordinate in some manner of the researcher, having to ask a direct question may exert undue influence and make it difficult, if not impossible, for the person to refuse to participate in a study. This would violate the principle of voluntary participation.

Informed Consent Form

In some cases the need for an informed consent form signed by the study participant may be waived. Studies that involve no risk to the subject may receive such waiver, especially if an informed consent form would unduly complicate the study or would affect the potential to recruit subjects. For example, when evaluating information systems to improve health literacy, persons with limited (health) literacy are the best subjects to recruit since they are the target population. However, having an extra document with information to read would pose an extra obstacle and may deter them from consenting to participate.

It is important that the informed consent form, and any other accompanying documentation, is evaluated for readability. The purpose of the form is to explain the study to potential participants. As mentioned above, before consent can be given, it is necessary for the person to understand that information. In the medical field, studies have shown that millions of people do not have sufficient health literacy to understand treatments or preventive care [8, 9]. As a result, it can be expected that these patients will not easily understand informed consent forms. It is therefore essential that researchers take this into account when conducting studies. The researcher should write the information as much as possible in layman's terms.

Writing the information in an understandable manner for laypersons is not easy. In medicine, the use of readability formulas is very popular to estimate the difficulty of text. The text is rewritten until an acceptable readability level has been achieved. The readability formulas that are used are metrics intended to describe the difficulty level of text. The most commonly used formula is the Flesch-Kincaid formula [10, 11] which estimates the readability level of a text using average syllable and word counts of sentences in the text. The formula provides a numeric evaluation of a text that represents the grade the reader should have completed in school to understand the text. For example, text can be written at an 8th grade level.

The researcher may consider applying readability formulas to this text, and some institutions may even require their researchers to use these formulas and write text at the 6th or 8th grade level, the recommended level for patient educational materials according to the American Medical Association [12]. However, the researcher should keep in mind that a low grade level is no guarantee for an easy-to-understand text. Very few studies using text on medical topics have shown a demonstrated improvement in understanding as a result of writing at low grade levels only. One exception is a study, which used the Cloze measure [13], a procedure where the nth word is deleted and participants need to fill in the blanks [14]. Furthermore, texts can easily be manipulated to lower the readability level, for example, by shortening the sentences, without any effect on readability or understanding. It is therefore better to conduct an evaluation of the consent form by representative participants as part of a pilot study. A teach-back method, where the participant explains the materials in the consent form to the researcher, will provide a good indication of how well the material was understood. There are no automated methods to estimate text difficulty as it would affect actual understanding [15–19].

When an informed consent form is required, it is part of the IRB documentation and needs to be approved by the IRB. It cannot be changed afterward without applying for approval of the changes. Not acquiring such consent, especially when critical or influential information is removed or added, may lead to criminal charges. Although such cases are rare, LeBlang [20] narrates the example of an ophthalmologist who removed language from an informed consent form indicating that a lens to be used in a cataract operation was still under clinical investigation. Participants were not informed this was an experimental procedure. A patient entered a lawsuit against several parties, including the hospital, medical device manufacturers and the ophthalmologist. The medical device manufacturers and the ophthalmologist entered into settlement agreements but the discussion about liability of the IRB continued in the courts.

Informed Consent Process

Several aspects of a study or participant characteristics may influence the consent process and the subjects' final decision to participate. Because of this complex nature, careful consideration is needed for the process itself. First of all, the researcher should realize that the location where the acquiring of informed consent takes place may unduly influence people's decision. This needs to be avoided. For example, requesting participation in a study while the person is in the doctor's office and the doctor is present would not be a good choice. The patient may feel obliged to consent. Furthermore, the location is important when discussing sensitive data. It is best to have a quiet, neutral and private area to explain the study. For example, personal information should not be discussed at the person's work or in public settings where others can overhear the conversation. Naturally, there are many studies that do not require these extra limitations. For example, evaluating a new search visualization algorithm does not require a private setting for the consent process, although the study itself probably will require such a setting so that subjects are not disturbed during their participation.

There are three groups of participants that require special consideration for the informed consent process. These are children and minors, adults with limited mental capacity and prisoners. All three groups may not have the capacity to understand the study and consent. Children and minors are not able to legally consent to participate in a study and informed consent will be needed from their parents or legal guardians. However, even when participants do not clearly belong to these three groups, the researcher should provide special treatment for any group of study participants who can be considered vulnerable subjects. For example, in many cases consent and participation cannot be given freely by people with temporarily limited cognitive abilities due to medication or disabilities.

Finally, payment of participants or providing other benefits, such as access to the latest treatments, devices or systems, may influence the voluntary consent. When participants are desperate to have access to the benefit provided by the study, they may see participation as their only possible option. Such benefits should be a special consideration when recruiting participants because, especially in medicine, those who are uninsured will be influenced by the perceived benefits.

Effects of IRB on Research

There has been much discussion about the optimal composition of an IRB, the research experience required of IRB members, how to make the process efficient and the role in and impact of IRB review on research. In a review conducted in 2001–2002 [21], based on a sample of approximately 3,000 researchers, it was shown that 11% of respondents had served on an IRB in the 3 years before the survey. This survey also showed that almost all serving members were active researchers. Having experienced researchers on the IRB will help ensure that they can provide a valuable evaluation. However, it may be worrying that almost half had consulted for industry during that period. In addition, having active researchers on the board may pose additional obstacles when evaluating competitive research or when there is a conflict of interest.

The IRB members usually are not trained IRB professionals but volunteers or faculty members required to do service for their university. As a result, the comments and requirements offered by the boards at different institutions may vary, even for the same study. Dyrbye et al. [22] compared six IRB applications for the same study at institutions associated with different medical schools. They found different requests, comments, and requirements and timelines. Naturally, this affects the efficiency with which research can be conducted at a particular institution. Being aware of who is on the board and what the review timeline is will help the researcher submit an application that will gain approval.

While the IRB protects study volunteers, the rules that are applied and the requirements dictated by the IRB are not without consequences. In particular, the requirement for written informed consent may affect the number of participants willing to participate, result in a bias of the study sample and slow down a study. It has been shown that these rules often influence which participants will participate and even which studies are conducted. For example, when working with consumers with very limited (health) literacy who visited soup kitchens, Miller [23] found it nearly impossible to have any participate in a study when it required a signed informed consent form. The invited participants were very suspicious of giving their name to anybody who 'looked official'. A systematic literature review by Kho et al. [24] showed such effects are not rare. They found that requiring written consent instigates a selection bias.

The roots of the IRB can be found several decades ago. The process helps ensure safety of humans who take part in experimentation. An IRB process has consequences for research though, and care should be taken that the original intent of such review and the common sense that is advocated also is maintained in informatics.

References

1. Dunn CM, Chadwick GL (2004) Protecting study volunteers in research: a manual for investigative sites, 3rd edn. Thomson Centerwatch, Boston
2. Baumrind D, Milgram S (2010) Classic dialogue: was Stanley Milgram's study of obedience unethical? In: Slife B (ed) Clashing views on psychological issues. McGraw-Hill, New York, pp 26–42
3. Milgram S (1963) Behavioral study of obedience. J Abnorm Soc Psychol 67(4):371–378
4. Garfinkel SL, Cranor LF (2010) Institutional review boards and your research: a proposal for improving the review procedures for research projects that involve human subjects and their associated identifiable private information. Commun ACM 53(6):38–40
5. Macklin R (2008) How independent are IRBs? IRB Ethics Hum Res 30(3):15–19
6. Hilgartner S (1990) Research fraud, misconduct, and the IRB. IRB Ethics Hum Res 12(1):1–4
7. Scheessele MR (2010) CS expertise for institutional review boards. ACM Comput 53(8):7
8. Committee on Health Literacy – Institute of Medicine of the National Academies (ed) (2004) Health literacy: a prescription to end confusion. The National Academies Press, Washington
9. Tokuda Y, Doba N, Butler JP, Paasche-Orlow MK (2009) Health literacy and physical and psychological wellbeing in Japanese adults. Patient Educ Couns 75(3):411–417
10. Flesch R (1948) A new readability yardstick. J Appl Psychol 32(3):221–233
11. Thomas G, Hartley RD, Kincaid JP (1975) Test-retest and inter-analyst reliability of the automated readability index, Flesch reading ease score, and the fog count. J Reading Behav 7(2):149–154
12. Weis BD (2007) Health literacy and patient safety: help patients understand. Manual for clinicians, 2nd edn. AMA and AMA Foundation, Chicago
13. Taylor WL (1953) Cloze procedure: a new tool for measuring readability. Journalism Q 30:415–433
14. Trifiletti LB, Shields WC, McDonald EM, Walker AR, Gielen AC (2006) Development of injury prevention materials for people with low literacy skills. Patient Educ Couns 64(1–3):119–127
15. Leroy G (2008) Improving health literacy with information technology. In: Wickramasinghe N, Geisler N (eds) Encyclopaedia of healthcare information systems. Idea Group, Inc., Information Science Reference, Hershey
16. Leroy G, Eryilmaz E, Laroya BT (2006) Health information text characteristics. In: American Medical Informatics Association (AMIA) annual symposium, Washington DC, 11–15 November 2006
17. Leroy G, Helmreich S, Cowie J (2010) The influence of text characteristics on perceived and actual difficulty of health information. Int J Med Inform 79(6):438–449
18. Leroy G, Helmreich S, Cowie JR (2010) The effects of linguistic features and evaluation perspective on perceived difficulty of medical text. In: Hawaii International Conference on System Sciences (HICSS), Kauai, 5–8 January 2010

19. Leroy G, Helmreich S, Cowie JR, Miller T, Zheng W (2008) Evaluating online health information: beyond readability formulas. In: AMIA, Washington DC, 8–12 November 2008
20. LeBlang TR (1995) Medical battery and failure to obtain informed consent: Illinois Court decision suggests potential for IRB liability. IRB Ethics Hum Res 17(3):10–11
21. Campbell EG, Weissman JS, Clarridge B, Yucel R, Causino N, Blumenthal D (2003) Characteristics of medical school faculty members serving on institutional review boards: results of a national survey. Acad Med 78(8):831–836
22. Dyrbye LN, Thomas MR, Mechaber AJ, Eacker A, Harper W, Massie FS Jr, Power DV, Shanafelt TD (2007) Medical education research and IRB review: an analysis and comparison of the IRB review process at six institutions. Acad Med 82:654–660
23. Miller T (2008) Dynamic generation of a health topics overview from consumer health information documents and its effect on user understanding, memory, and recall. Doctoral Dissertation, Claremont Graduate University, Claremont
24. Kho ME, Duffett M, Willison D, Cook DJ, Brouwers MC (2009) Written informed consent and selection bias in observational studies using medical records: systematic review. BMJ 338:b866

Resources

12

Chapter Summary

This chapter provides an overview of resources available to developers and researchers who intend to evaluate their information systems systematically with human participants. The chapter starts by describing pilot studies. Although many would not think of this as a resource per se, conducting pilot studies is invaluable. It allows for evaluation of the final study design and also will provide valuable feedback on the system itself. It is therefore emphasized in this section. Next, several existing resources are described such as test data and gold standards, vocabularies and more structured knowledge sources such as ontologies. A few data analysis tools are also highlighted.

This chapter does not attempt to provide a final and conclusive list since new resources are made available every day. However, an attempt is made here to highlight resources that have particular value or that are not usually referred to in existing manuals and textbooks. The focus is on those that are available or provide a version that is available as open source or for free. The resources are ordered alphabetically. For more open source software, the reader is referred to SourceForge (http://sourceforge.net/). The reader should note that free usage is typically reserved for researchers and nonprofit organizations.

Pilot Studies as Resources

Information systems are developed over several cycles. Early on, the basic functionality is evaluated to ensure no errors are made, that input and output are correct and that the program runs in reasonable time using reasonable memory resources. Depending on how the system was designed and how much involvement there was from the intended users in the initial phases, the mental model that the developers will have of the system's required functionality will be much different from that of the intended users. In very few cases will the two mental models be identical. An exception is usually found when users and developers are the same group of people.

G. Leroy, *Designing User Studies in Informatics*, Health Informatics,
DOI 10.1007/978-0-85729-622-1_12, © Springer-Verlag London Limited 2011

However, since developers and intended users are typically very different, early and frequent pilot studies are necessary for success of the final product.

Regardless of the differences between developers and users, pilot studies are also necessary before conducting a full-scale user evaluation. This is especially the case in medicine, where access to users is often difficult, costly and time consuming. Conducting a pilot study will help avoid errors in the evaluation approach and will make it possible to fix problems, both in the evaluation and in the information system, early on. Moreover, it will impact planning the practical details of a study and many problems can be ironed out, especially if the evaluator is inexperienced. Before conducting a pilot study, the researcher or developer should check whether IRB approval is required. Some institutions do not consider pilot studies to be research and do not require IRB review; others require IRB review for any studies involving human subjects.

The closer a pilot study resembles the final study, the more valuable it will be. To show the potential of a study, to work out potential problems in advance and to make the best of an opportunity to make improvements, it is essential to conduct a pilot study as if it were the final study. This includes the process to recruit and sign up participants using the intended recruitment materials. Moreover, the study materials, conduct of the researcher, location of the study, reimbursement type and method, and any software to be used can be tested. The results of a pilot study will then be indicative of future results of the evaluation and may even reveal interesting effects.

The number of participants and the effect this has on the power of the study to detect significant effects is discussed in Chap. 3. An example suffices to illustrate the point. When a pilot study with few participants shows significance levels of the independent variable of $p = 0.09$ or even smaller, this is a first indication that with more participants, the effect of the independent variable will most likely be significant. In contrast, when the significance levels are much larger than 0.1 or when the study outcomes are not in the hypothesized direction, the researchers can draw early conclusions and may prefer to improve the information system before conducting the study. Naturally, the pilot study can only be used in this manner when it was conducted as a valid user study and care was taken not to introduce bias. Although a complete list of all advantages of a pilot study and all problems that can be found is impossible, below is a list of the advantages one can expect from pilot studies.

Time management is important in pilot studies and affects recruitment and retention of participants. The time needed by a participant to complete a study is difficult to estimate, especially when the participants have very different personal characteristics from the researchers, for example, when working with children or persons with mental disabilities. By conducting a pilot study, the researcher can get an estimate of the required time, get a first reaction to the system and furthermore get the participants' feedback on the meta-aspects of the study itself, for example, the difficulty level of tasks or the time required for completion. Knowing the test duration itself will also help with scheduling participants.

Practical skills will be gained when conducting a pilot study. This is especially important to ensure that all participants are treated in the same manner so that no bias is introduced. Instructions can be practiced and the researchers will gain experience guiding participants through the experimental condition. Although this may seem trivial, having objective instructions that are similar for all conditions is essential. When instructions differ between conditions, they may lead to confounding. When instructions differ within a condition, they will introduce additional error variance and reduce the power of the experiment.

Problems with the study materials can be caught early. These range from practical problems related to the instructions, which may be too complex or the font too small, to the use of inappropriate tasks, such as tasks that are irrelevant or unimportant to the users, and even the method to provide reimbursement receipts that complicates maintaining confidentiality. More fundamental problems with the study itself can also be caught. Surveys may be too general, too complicated or unsuitable for showing differences between conditions. For example, in a study to evaluate perceived text difficulty, Leroy et al. [1, 2] found that comparing too many grammatically different versions of a sentence resulted in nonsense data. Participants could not evaluate 16 different versions. The study was redesigned so that the subjects evaluated groups of four sentences instead. Metrics may turn out to be not sufficiently sensitive or the tasks may need to be better aligned with the intention of the study. For example, when comparing different user interfaces, some changes in the interface may go completely unnoticed by study participants when they are intent on completing a task not designed to test that aspect of the interface.

Data collection and analysis methods can be evaluated and tuned. Conducting the data analysis for pilot studies will be valuable in pointing out missing data or redundant data that does not contribute to the experiment. It may also impact how the final data will be collected to make it practical to objectively process and analyze results from a much larger group of participants than those who participated in the pilot study. This will also help estimate the time needed to analyze the data, which may be needed to schedule and budget outside evaluators.

Programmatically tracking data is a feature that is best evaluated in a pilot study. When information systems are evaluated, it is often convenient to add a tracking function so that user interactions, errors and use time can be tracked by the software without putting an additional burden on the study participants and without an observer being present. However, this adds more complexity to the information system since additional software components need to be integrated. Therefore, a short pilot study is very valuable in revealing program errors as well as missing data or inconsistencies. The pilot study can be used to verify if the tracked data coincides with the actual usage. For example, in a pilot study of communication software for children with autism [3, 4], communication behaviors were tracked during a longitudinal study. The children were taught by their teacher to use a mobile device to communicate. Their behavior was tracked for several weeks and subsequent data analysis showed two unexpected features. First, it showed that the mobile device was seldom turned off but put in hibernation mode instead, potentially leading to memory problems. Second, the time and date capturing was inconsistent: time was captured for every usage, while the date was captured only when the software was started. This made is impossible to calculate daily averages of use.

Datasets and Gold Standards

Text, Audio, Video and Other Corpora

The *Directory of Open Access Journals* (www.doaj.org) lists more than 5,000 open access journals of which more than 1,000 are related to healthcare, medicine or the life sciences. The idea for the directory originates back to the First Nordic Conference on Scholarly Communication in 2002 (Copenhagen) and was supported by the Open Society Foundations. The directory is currently hosted, maintained and partly funded by Lund University Libraries Head Office in Sweden.

The *Internet Archive* (http://www.archive.org/) is a nonprofit organization that provides a digital library of free online resources. It is not limited to medical websites. It came into existence in 1996 and has been adding information to its collection ever since. It includes music, audio, movies, software and text. The websites collected are not limited to English language sites; most languages are supported. What makes it unique is that it contains snapshots of Internet resources taken at different points in time that are all available. For example, a website can be revisited by typing in the URL using the WayBackMachine. If the website was included in the archive, its different versions over time are available. For example, the archive retains copies as far back as 1997 of the National Library of Medicine website.

The *Linguistic Data Consortium* (http://www.ldc.upenn.edu), founded in 1992, provides several different data collections, including speech and text databases, for example, public speeches or telephone conversations, training data and lexicons. The consortium members are universities, companies and research laboratories. The data collections are available to members, who pay an annual membership fee. Many of the resources can also be purchased by nonmembers. There are resources for a variety of different languages and on a variety of different topics. Several of the resources are relevant to biology and medicine. For example, there is the PennBioIE Ontology which contains annotated PubMed abstracts or BioProp which focuses on propositions in biomedical text.

The *MEDLINE* database contains millions of biomedical abstracts complete with structured meta-information such as author names, journal names, publication data, and Medical Subject Headings (MeSH). It can be downloaded from the National Library of Medicine. Researchers wanting to download it need to sign the license. The data can be downloaded via ftp or received on tape and is distributed in XML format. Information about the size, format, distribution, license and other related topics can be found on the website of the U.S. National Library of Medicine, under Bibliographic Services Division, MEDLINE®/PubMed® data. This site (http://www.nlm.nih.gov/bsd/licensee/medpmmenu.html) also provides the links to the pages where the dataset can be downloaded.

Ontologies, Thesauri and Lexicons

The *Consumer Health Vocabulary* (CHV) (www.consumerhealthvocab.org) is a resource containing consumer terms and their mappings to the Unified Medical

Language System (UMLS) terminology. It contains approximately 150,000 terms assigned to 60,000 UMLS concepts [5, 6]. Each term and concept has been assigned a score indicating its understandability to laypersons. A concept represents an underlying idea common to a set of terms. Understandability scores are based on frequency counts in large text corpora and range from 0 to 1, with a higher score representing better understandability. This resource also indicates if a word is a preferred description for a concept by the CHV or the UMLS.

Freebase (http://wiki.freebase.com) was originally developed by MetaWeb Technologies Inc., which was acquired by Google in 2010. It is a repository containing several millions of entities that are linked together in a graph; each entity forms a node and is linked to other nodes. There are dozens of topics and several are relevant to the medical domain. The resource is available under the Creative Commons Attribution License.

GALEN is technology used to represent medical information that produces a coding system. It uses the GALEN Common Reference Model which is intended to represent medical concepts in an application-independent but also language-independent manner. OpenGALEN (http://www.opengalen.org) is a nonprofit organization that provides (open source) licenses for the GALEN Common Reference Model.

The Weizman Institute, located in Israel, provides the *GeneCard* database (www.genecards.org) which contains data on known and predicted human genes. It integrates transcriptomic, genetic, proteomic, functional and disease information from different sources. The database can be searched online and a card is provided for each gene with detailed information, references and links to 3D images.

The *Gene Ontology* (http://www.geneontology.org/) is provided by the Gene Ontology Consortium and was initially formed by combining the model organisms for FlyBase (Drosophila), Saccharomyces and Mouse in 1998. The Gene Ontology contains three structured vocabularies that list gene products and terms for biological processes, cellular components and molecular functions. The information is now provided in a species neutral manner.

The *GENIA Corpus* (http://www-tsujii.is.s.u-tokyo.ac.jp/GENIA/) contains approximately 2,000 biomedical abstracts and was specifically created to support the development of biomedical text mining systems. It has been compiled and annotated within the scope of the GENIA project, the goal of which is to develop text mining systems for molecular biology. The abstracts are annotated with a variety of information, such as parts-of-speech, syntactic tree annotation, term annotation for genes, cells and proteins, biomedical events, relations, such as has-mutant, cellular localization and also relationship to diseases. Additional tools for Natural Language Processing (NLP) are also provided.

The *Medical Subject Headings (MeSH)* (http://www.nlm.nih.gov/mesh/) are provided by the U.S. National Library of Medicine (NLM). It is a controlled thesaurus containing a hierarchy of medical terms. The thesaurus dates back to 1960 and is used by the NLM to index the articles in the MEDLINE/PubMED®.

The U.S. *National Cancer Institute (NCI) Thesaurus* (http://ncit.nci.nih.gov/) contains the current vocabulary for clinical care, research activities in biomedicine and non-clinical but relevant terms related to administrative activities and public information. It is linked to the *NCI MetaThesaurus* (http://ncim.nci.nih.gov/ncimbrowser) and together they provide over 3,600,000 terms and the 1,400,000 biomedical concepts that represent their meaning. They also provide more than 200,000 cross links between terms, preferred terms, synonyms and definitions.

The *Unified Medical Language Systems* (*UMLS*, www.nlm.nih.gov) is also provided by the NLM. It is a collection of thesauri available to the research community. It has three components. The Metathesaurus contains terms, concepts representing underlying meaning for the terms and semantic types. The Semantic Network contains the semantic types and the relations between them. The Specialist Lexicon is a linguistic resource for English containing words, spelling variants and parts of speech.

An extensive list with links to biomedical and biological ontologies is provided by the *Open Biological and Biomedical Ontologies Foundry* [7] (http://www.obofoundry.org/). Additional ontologies can be developed using *Protégé* (http://protege.stanford.edu/), an open source ontology development tool. Furthermore, there exist several resources not specifically created for medicine but that nevertheless may be useful for the development or evaluation of information systems for healthcare, medicine and biology.

Cyc (http://www.cyc.com/) is a knowledge base containing machine readable common sense knowledge. Portions of the ontology, called *openCyc* (http://opencyc.org/), have been made publicly and freely available. This portion contains hundreds of thousands of terms and millions of relations between the terms. The Cyc Foundation (http://www.cycfoundation.org) aims to expand and enrich this free resource and promote its utilization among developers.

FrameNet [8] (http://framenet.icsi.berkeley.edu/) focuses on frame semantics. It provides almost 1,000 frames with more than 150,000 annotated sentences to illustrate the frames. The goal is to show the semantic and syntactic options for different meanings, called senses, of words.

The *Google Corpus*, created by Google and available from the Linguistic Data Consortium (http://www.ldc.upenn.edu), contains n-grams for its collection of text. An n-gram is a sequence of *n* words. Google processed 1,024,908,267,229 tokens and calculated the frequency of all unigrams, bigrams, trigrams, fourgrams and five-grams in the corpus.

WordNet [9] (http://wordnet.princeton.edu), developed at Princeton, is a general English lexical resource containing both semantic and syntactic information organized in cognitive synonyms, called synsets, for English language nouns, verbs, adjectives and adverbs. The synsets are linked by conceptual-semantic and lexical relations. Over the years, different versions have been developed in dozens of languages, which can be reviewed from the site of the Global WordNet Association (www.globalwordnet.org).

Gold Standards

The *Text REtrieval Conference* (*TREC*) (http://trec.nist.gov/) was co-sponsored by the National Institute of Standards and Technology (NIST) and the U.S. Department of Defense. For several years starting in 1992, the conference provided researchers with datasets, tasks and answers to the tasks. The goal was to develop algorithms for information retrieval and compare them using the same tasks and evaluation approaches. There are many tracks on different topics, and a genomics track was included from 2003 to 2007. Most data collections, including the tasks and answers, are available online or can be requested.

The U.S. National Library of Medicine provides a small collection useful for training algorithms for *word sense disambiguation* (http://wsd.nlm.nih.gov/). Word senses refer to the multiple meanings that many words have. To disambiguate the different senses, the context of the word and understanding that context is needed. Machine learning algorithms are typically used to do this automatically. The provided collection contains 50 UMLS concepts. For each concept, there are 100 instances selected and disambiguated. The disambiguation was conducted by a team of 11 experts.

Data Gathering, Storage and Analysis Tools

Collecting User Responses

Amazon's Mechanical Turk (https://www.mturk.com/) is an online service that can be used by researchers and study participants. Both groups first need to sign up with the service. Researchers can compose small tasks that can be completed online and they provide payment for completing the task. Subjects choose tasks to work on and receive payment for participating in multiple studies.

Survey Monkey (www.surveymonkey.com) is an online tool that can be used for free or for a fee. The free version has a limitation on the number and type of questions that can be posed and also on the ease with which analysis can be done. The tool is very easy to use and an online survey can be composed in a matter of minutes, not counting the time it takes to design the statements, of course. Respondents use the Internet to complete the survey and the data can be analyzed in detail.

Databases

While there are many databases and data storage options available for sale, there are also an increasing number of resources made available for free. These include the smaller or educational versions of databases such as Oracle and Microsoft SQL Server and also an increasing list of open source databases. Below is a short list of open source databases. They may be more or less developed (key-value stores and relational models) and scalable:
- Apache Cassandra: http://cassandra.apache.org/.
- Apache Derby: http://db.apache.org/derby/.
- CouchDB: http://couchdb.apache.org/.
- Daffodil: http://db.daffodilsw.com/.

- Firebird: http://www.firebirdsql.org/.
- Hadoop: http://hadoop.apache.org/, several database products.
- Hypertable: http://www.hypertable.org/.
- mongoDB: http://www.mongodb.org/.
- MySQL: http://www.mysql.com/, the community edition is available as a free and open source product.
- Neo4j: http://neo4j.org/, a graph database.
- PostgreSQL: http://www.postgresql.org/.
- Redis: http://code.google.com/p/redis/.
- Riak: http://www.basho.com/Riak.html.
- SQLite: http://www.sqlite.org/.

Data Analysis

Weka is a suite of machine learning algorithms, written in Java, for classification, clustering, association and visualization. All algorithms can be combined with evaluation components, such as accuracy confusion matrices or n-fold cross-validation evaluation. Information on its algorithms and usage is available in an accompanying book by Witten and Frank [10]. The toolkit can be downloaded from http://www.cs.waikato.ac.nz/ml/weka/.

More data mining tools are described and available from http://www.kdnuggets.com/.

Other

GATE (http://gate.ac.uk/) is open source natural language processing (NLP) software, written in Java, developed at the University of Sheffield's Department of Computer Science. It provides a flexible framework that allows developers to build new and fine-tune existing components [11]. Several components are provided that can be combined into a pipeline and then applied to text. Additional components can be developed and integrated with the existing components. The new components are usually written as a Java Annotation Patterns Engine (JAPE). These are text files containing rules typically used for annotating terms or chunks of text. There is a large user community and several new resources, for example, plugins for WordNet, are being made available.

The National Library of Medicine offers additional developer resources as part of its *Semantic Knowledge Representation* (http://skr.nlm.nih.gov). These are available for use by developers who sign the UMLS license. Users can schedule batch jobs which use internal components such as MetaMap and SemRep [12] to map natural language text in English to semantic predications and the associated UMLS components. Academic papers describing the components are also available. For example, SemRep's precision has been estimated at 83% for the ISA predication [12] and ranging from 53% to 92% for other predications [13, 14].

Guidelines, Certification, Training and Credits

A *Certificate of Confidentiality* is issued in the U.S. to protect study participants' information. Researchers conducting human subjects research can apply for a certificate when the study involves collecting information about study participants that may harm participants if the information were made public or disclosed. The certificate protects against legal requests for this information. Details can be found at the Certificates of Confidentiality Kiosk (http://grants.nih.gov/grants/policy/coc/).

There are several resources with advice on how to write easy-to-read versions of healthcare-related text suitable for reading by laypersons. MedlinePlus (http://www.nlm.nih.gov/medlineplus/etr.html) provides guidelines for writing easy-to-read health information. The National Institutes of Health (NIH) has its more general The Plain Language Initiative (http://execsec.od.nih.gov/plainlang/index.html), the state of California has the California Health Literacy initiative (http://cahealthliteracy.org/) and others such as the Health & Literacy Special Collection (http://lincs.worlded.org/) also provide advice.

Some research institutions require *Human Subjects Study Certification* of their researchers before they can conduct research with human subjects. Although this is seldom the case for researchers in information and computer science who evaluate algorithms, it is often so for researchers in medicine or genomics. Many institutions have their own requirements, while others rely on outside resources. For example, a certificate in protecting human study subjects can be earned from:

- The National Institutes of Health offer online courses (http://phrp.nihtraining.com) that are free to take and an interesting read. After completion, a certificate is provided and kept on file.
- CME or AMA PRA Category 1 Credits or nursing contact hours can be earned for completing the exam associated with the manual "Protecting Study Volunteers in Research" [15]. This book also contains a detailed section relevant to genomics research and working with individuals and their genomic information. The answers to the exam are mailed and graded by The University of Rochester School of Medicine and Dentistry, which is accredited by the Accreditation Council for Continuing Medical Education and provides continuing medical education for physicians.

Protection of Human Subjects

A copy of the *Belmont Report* can be obtained online (http://www.hhs.gov/ohrp/belmontArchive.html) together with associated guidelines at: www.hhs.gov/ohrp/humansubjects/guidance/belmont.htm.

Central IRB (CIRB) (www.ncicirb.org) focuses on cancer-related research. The Central Institutional Review Board of the National Cancer Institute (NCI) of the National Institutes of Health (NIH) is an initiative started in 2001 to help lighten the load of local IRBs. Membership is at the institutional level.

Declaration of Helsinki: http://www.wma.net/en/30publications/10policies/b3/index.html.

Nuremberg Code: http://ohsr.od.nih.gov/guidelines/nuremberg.html.

U.S. *HIPAA Privacy Rule*: http://www.hhs.gov/ocr/privacy/index.html.

U.S. *Protection of Human Subjects* provides information about research that is exempt, expedited or requires a full review at http://www.hhs.gov/ohrp/humansubjects/guidance/45cfr46.htm, with more details on expedited review at http://www.hhs.gov/ohrp/humansubjects/guidance/expedited98.htm.

Commercial entities providing an IRB:

- The *Association for the Accreditation of Human Research Protection Program* (AAHRPP) (http://www.aahrpp.org) is a for-profit organization that provides accreditation to institutions across the world. It is not limited to the United States. Institutions submit to the review process on a voluntary basis. This group's goal is to work with the research organizations and accredit them to do their research with humans. The accreditation itself is based on a review of policies, procedures and practices to ensure sound research and protection of human rights. The accreditation process starts with a self-evaluation, followed by a site visit which leads to a report by the organization within a month. The submitting organization has the option to reply to the report, and final accreditation is based on this inter-action. The first accreditation is granted for 3 years and subsequent re-accreditations are for 5 years. Since this is a for-profit organization, organizations pay an application fee and an annual fee thereafter.
- *Biomedical Research Alliance of New York* (BRANY) (http://www.brany.com), is sponsored by over 200 companies, many of them pharmaceuticals and biotech companies. The group works together with many hospitals, research centers, clinics and other types of research groups. They offer several services, including IRB reviews, for a fee, while other services, such as support with site selection for studies, are provided for free.
- The *Western Institutional Review Board* (WIRB) (http://www.wirb.com) is a for-profit organization that provides reviews of research involving human subjects for individual researchers and for institutions around the world. There is no expedited review for any initial review of research but the institute does provide IRB determination of exemptions. It expects researchers to show evidence of training in human subjects research that goes beyond simple experience.

Professional Organizations with additional resources and guidelines:

- American Medical Association (AMA), http://www.ama-assn.org/.
- American Psychological Association (APA), http://www.apa.org/.
- European Federation of Psychologist's Associations (EFPA), http://www.efpa.eu/.

References

1. Leroy G, Helmreich S, Cowie J (2010) The influence of text characteristics on perceived and actual difficulty of health information. Int J Med Inform 79(6):438–449

2. Leroy G, Helmreich S, Cowie JR (2010) The effects of linguistic features and evaluation perspective on perceived difficulty of medical text. In: Hawaii international conference on system sciences (HICSS), Kauai, 5–8 January 2010

3. De Leo G, Gonzales C, Battagiri P, Leroy G (2010) A smart-phone application and a companion website for the improvement of the communication skills of children with autism: clinical rationale, technical development and preliminary results. J Med Syst. DOI: 10.1007/s10916-009-9407-1

4. Leroy G, Chuang S, Huang J, Charlop-Christy MJ (2005) Digital libraries on handhelds for autistic children. In: ACM I (ed) Fifth ACM + IEEE joint conference on digital libraries (JCDL-2005), Denver, Colorado, 7–11 June 2005

5. Zeng QT, Tse T, Crowell J, Divita G, Roth L, Browne AC (2005) Identifying consumer-friendly display (CFD) names for health concepts. In: AMIA 2005 fall symposium, Washington DC, USA, 2005, pp 859–863

6. Keselman A, Smith CA, Divita G, Kim H, Browne A, Leroy G, Zeng-Treitler Q (2008) Consumer health concepts that do not map to the UMLS: where do they fit? J Am Med Inform Assoc 15(4):496–505

7. Smith B, Ashburner M, Rosse C, Bard C, Bug W, Ceusters W, Goldberg LJ, Eilbeck K, Ireland A, Mungall CJ, The OBI Consortium, Leontis N, Rocca-Serra P, Ruttenberg A, Sansone S-A, Scheuermann RH, Shah N, Whetzel PL, Lewis S (2007) The OBO Foundry: coordinated evolution of ontologies to support biomedical data integration. Nat Biotechnol 25:251–1255

8. Fillmore CJ, Baker CF (2010) A frame approach to semantic analysis. In: Heine B, Narrog H (eds) Oxford handbook of linguistic analysis. OUP

9. Miller GA, Beckwidth R, Fellbaum C, Gross D, Miller K (1998) Introduction to WordNet: an on-line lexical database. http://www.cogsci.princeton.edu/~wn

10. Witten IH, Frank E (2000) Data mining: practical machine learning tools and techniques with Java. The Morgan Kaufmann Series in data management systems. Morgan Kaufmann, San Francisco

11. Cunningham H, Maynard D, Bontcheva K, Tablan V (2002) GATE: a framework and graphical development environment for robust NLP tools and applications. In: 40th Anniversary Meeting of the Association for Computational Linguistics (ACL'02), Philadelphia, July 2002

12. Rindflesch TC, Fiszman M (2003) The interaction of domain knowledge and linguistic structure in natural language processing: interpreting hypernymic propositions in biomedical text. J Biomed Inform 36(6):462–477

13. Rindflesch TC, Libbus B, Hristovski D, Aronson AR, Kilicoglu H (2003) Semantic relations asserting the etiology of genetic diseases. In: AMIA annual symposium, 2003, pp 554–558

14. Fiszman M, Rindflesch TC, Kilicoglu H (2004) Abstraction summarization for managing the biomedical research literature. In: Workshop on Computational Lexical Semantics (HLT-NAACL), 2004, pp 76–83

15. Dunn CM, Chadwick GL (2004) Protecting study volunteers in research: a manual for investigative sites, 3rd edn. Thomson Centerwatch Inc, Boston

Part III

Common Mistakes to Avoid

Avoid Bias

13

Chapter Summary

In previous chapters, nuisance variables and the biases they may bring about were discussed. It is vital to the study that such bias is avoided. This chapter provides an overview of several countermeasures that can be taken. This section discusses errors that can be avoided after which the study designs are greatly improved, often without increasing the cost or time it takes to complete the studies.

Subject-related bias, where the subjects' behavior is different from what could be expected in normal circumstances, can be countered in many ways, ranging from increasing the neutrality of the location to conducting a single-blind study where subjects do not know to which experimental condition they are assigned. Experimenter-related bias, where the experimenter unintentionally influences the study results or the subjects, can be countered with measures ranging from standardized instructions and behaviors to using a double-blind approach where both subjects and experimenter do not know to which experimental condition the subject is assigned. Design-related bias, where scores or behaviors change because of the manner in which conditions are carried out or ordered, can be countered with measures ranging from simple time delays to counterbalanced ordering of treatments to even out potential bias. Naturally, designing a user study involves trade-offs and the researcher should be careful that countering one type of bias does not introduce another.

Countermeasures for Subject-Related Bias

Subject-related bias is the result of subjects acting a certain way because they know they are participating in a study. In general, this bias can be reduced or avoided if participants do not have the opportunity to develop a loyalty or antipathy for the researchers and their work. There are several specific countermeasures that can be taken, some of which are easier to accomplish than others. The following is a list of examples of what can be done. This is by no means an exhaustive list, and there are no easy approaches to choosing which countermeasures to incorporate.

G. Leroy, *Designing User Studies in Informatics*, Health Informatics,
DOI 10.1007/978-0-85729-622-1_13, © Springer-Verlag London Limited 2011

The *location of the experiment* may lead to bias, for example, when a study is conducted in a clinical setting, a laboratory or a hospital the participating subjects may feel intimidated and may not act normally. This unintended effect may be reinforced if a clinician conducts the study because this person might be seen as an authority figure by the participants. A neutral location, if possible, will help avoid the associated bias and may also improve recruitment and retention of participants since it may be possible to choose a convenient location for subjects. However, care should be taken that no other types of bias are introduced by changing the location. For example, conducting the study in a public environment may require dealing with noise and distractions. Similarly, conducting the study at home may lead to other interruptions, for example, by small children or pets. These variations will increase error variance in the study.

Explaining the importance of honesty and fulfilling the task as requested is another tactic that may be helpful. In order to please the experimenter participants may change their behavior, answers or opinions. Making it clear to all participants that lying or acting differently helps nobody (this may counter the altruism bias) and actually decreases (or negates) the value of their contribution (this may counter the look good bias) will help avoid such bias.

Limiting the interaction of the participant with the researcher should also be considered. When there are many interactions, participants may develop an opinion about the experimenter herself. For example, they may especially like the experimenter or, on the other hand, they may develop an antipathy for her. Each situation would most probably affect the study. If interaction cannot be limited, a good option is to employ a facilitator for the study. This is a person who interacts with the participants but is not the researcher herself. If such a distinction can be made, participants should be told about it. The informed consent form, if used, can include this information. Keep in mind that such facilitators should be trained. If multiple facilitators are employed in the study, they should all be trained in the same manner. One should be careful not to assign a different facilitator to each experimental condition, since this would then be a confounded variable with the independent variable: it would be impossible to know whether effects are due to the treatment or the facilitator. Therefore, ensure that facilitators lead different conditions (preferably all) and, if possible, that they are not aware of which condition they are leading (see double blinding later in this section).

Providing anonymity or *confidentiality* may further help avoid subject-related bias. People may feel freer to act and react when they know that their answers will not be associated with their personal information. This approach may be strengthened by using a facilitator since then the answers will not be evaluated or judged by the person with whom the participants interact. Naturally, this will only work when participants are informed about this and precautions similar to those explained above are taken.

A *single-blind controlled* study (double-blind is discussed in the next section) is an experimental control where participants are not aware of which experimental condition they are participating in. If participants partake in all experimental conditions, they should be unaware of which condition they are participating in at a particular time. This helps control bias due to knowledge of the experimental treatment. For example, the expectations will be different for experimental conditions and control conditions which may cloud many measurements. For some studies in informatics, this may be difficult to accomplish. For example, when a new and an old system are compared for current users, the participants in the study will have experience using the old system and will clearly see which condition is which. Moreover, they may have opinions about each even before the start of the study. When multiple versions of a new system are being compared, single blinding can be achieved more easily.

Making the user tasks realistic is also helpful. It will help participants focus on the tasks instead of spending time guessing about the goals and measurements of the study. In informatics, realistic tasks provide the additional advantage that both objective and subjective measures can be used and compared. For example, success and error rates can be calculated. When both the objective and subjective measures show the same results, little bias was introduced. However, sometimes the researcher will find that the objective measures tell a different story from the subjective measures. For example, when comparing a new information system to an existing baseline, subjects may indicate that they prefer the new system while objective measures show no difference between the two systems. This difference may be due to a real preference or, if no countermeasures were taken, to bias.

Finally, *taking into account a possible variety of participant characteristics* when designing the study may lead to a different and better study design. It may affect the dependent variable chosen for the study. For example, when measuring understanding or learning, the background knowledge and previously studied materials may influence the scores on the dependent variable. Not distinguishing between participants with different starting levels of knowledge would make these scores too coarse to interpret. A pre- and post-intervention comparison of understanding would provide a better measurement of the effect of the intervention. Taking user characteristics into account may also change the study procedures, and, for example, training may be included when it is suspected that participants have different levels of expertise with a system or do not possess the necessary technical skills. For example, when developing software for children with autism, Leroy et al. [1] found that the technical skills of special education teachers influenced the results of the pilot studies; some subjects did not understand how to open and save compressed files (.zip) and required training to do this.

Countermeasures for Experimenter-Related Bias

Experimenter-related bias refers to effects that are the result of experimenter behaviors. In general, many experimenter-related effects can be more or less avoided by having multiple evaluators, by training the evaluators and controlling their behavior, by providing a clear gold standard in advance and by using double-blind study designs. As in the previous section, the following is a list of possible countermeasures to be considered by the researcher.

Providing a professional and courteous interaction will help avoid counter effects due to personal characteristics. This requires the researcher to look professional and adopt a professional attitude. It will help avoid subject-related bias as described above.

Standardizing the instructions is important. All participants should receive their instructions in the same manner. Experimenters or facilitators should practice their interaction with participants. If the experiment is conducted in a language other than the facilitator's native language, the facilitator should practice giving the instructions and answering questions.

Using multiple facilitators helps reduce experimenter effects if they exist so that any bias will be less systematic. In addition, a study effect that is repeated regardless of who the facilitator was allows for a stronger conclusion since the result is more general. An important additional advantage of working with facilitators is that it is easier to achieve a double-blind condition (see below). Naturally, adding more facilitators to run the experiment requires that all are trained in the same manner. It is best to train them together so they receive the same instructions and practice. They could observe each other during pilot studies to help standardize their behavior. It may be helpful to observe the facilitators since more standardized behavior can be expected from facilitators who know they are being observed. When there are multiple facilitators and experimental conditions, the facilitators should be distributed across the different conditions. A balance should be sought in the number of facilitators since working with multiple facilitators will require more resources and will also lead to a more complex study design.

Reducing the influence of the facilitator or experimenter will lower the potential for bias and make it easier to achieve a double-blind condition. When there is little interaction, the facilitator will have less opportunity to observe or deduce the experimental conditions. Especially in informatics studies, this option can be more easily achieved when the instructions, explanations and tasks are conveyed by computer. Limiting the role of the facilitator to welcoming and reimbursing subjects will remove bias. On the other hand, it may reduce the participants' effort since there is little personal interaction. Another potential bias to be taken into account is that of training over time. Facilitators who have been part of the study for a longer time and have worked with multiple subjects will have a different interaction style than those with less experience. It may also be beneficial to consider the facilitators as an explicitly controlled nuisance variable and to calculate the existence of an effect, if any.

Using a double-blind condition will further reduce bias. In many cases the researcher, facilitator or developer will be biased toward a specific condition. To avoid this, an experiment can be conducted in double-blind fashion when both the subject and facilitator are blind to the experimental condition. Similar to single-blind studies, the participants are not aware which treatment they are receiving. A double-blind control can be achieved by ensuring the experimenter also does not know the treatment condition.

A double-blind condition is difficult to achieve in informatics studies since the information system that is being developed usually is easy to recognize and identify. Nearly double-blind evaluations can be accomplished with the creation and use of a gold standard for evaluation. The results of applying the information system or algorithm can be compared against that gold standard. For example, the author used the gold standard approach when developing the algorithms that were part of a biomedical search engine. An expert tagged several biomedical texts to indicate the relevant entities in the text. The outcome of information extraction algorithms was then compared against the gold standard. A similar approach is accomplished when the outcomes from different conditions are randomized and then evaluated by an expert, instead of compared against a gold standard, who does not know the origin of each result. For example, when evaluating the outcome of different search engines, the results for each condition can be combined in one results list (without duplicates). Experts or representative users can review this entire list, resulting in a double-blind evaluation of the outcome. Once this has been completed, the scores for the individual abstracts can be traced back to the experimental condition.

Countermeasures for Design-Related Bias

Several biases can be introduced by the use of a particular experimental design. Especially with within-subjects designs, subjects participate in multiple conditions which may lead to biases related to the order of conditions or experience gained during the experiment. With between-subjects designs, the bias is generally related to the experimenter and differences between conditions and the countermeasures for this have been discussed above.

Using a crossover design is helpful in controlling carryover effects and ordering effects. Carryover effects or contamination effects are found when effects from the control condition carry over to the experimental condition. Ordering effects are the result of having multiple experimental conditions. To avoid or control both types of problems, the order of conditions should be counterbalanced. For example, if there are two conditions, the order needs to be reversed for half of the participants. If there is a carryover effect, a different result would be found in the second group compared to the first group. By changing the order for half of the participants, the effects cancel out if they exist. In addition, by systematically reversing the order for half the participants, it is possible to explicitly verify whether there was a carryover effect. When there are more than 2 conditions, the order can be counterbalanced in a similar manner. For example, a group in the Netherlands evaluated 2 versions of the Well-being Questionnaire (WBQ) and the Diabetes Treatment Satisfaction Questionnaire (DTSQ) using a crossover design [2]. They found that the paper-based and computer-based versions were equivalent but also demonstrated a carryover effect of some of the subscales, namely for depression and energy scales. Leroy et al. [3] used a within-subjects design to evaluate 5 search engine algorithms for query augmentation. Since people could become better with practice or worse due to fatigue, different possible orderings of the algorithms were used. This difference in order was unknown to the subjects. By evaluating performance by experimental condition and also by the order in which it was executed, it was shown that the performance of the subjects was not due to the order but due to a difference in the underlying algorithms.

Leaving sufficient time between experimental conditions may help avoid a carryover effect and also a second look bias. Second look bias is the result of interacting multiple times with the information system under different experimental conditions. Unfortunately, leaving enough time in between conditions is not always practical or possible. Moreover, when there is too much time in between experimental conditions, other events may happen (history effect) and influence the outcome. If a time delay is not an option, the bias can be avoided by executing a between-subjects design instead of a within-subjects design by not reusing the information system. In informatics, the second look principle also applies to a second look at data or user tasks. When study participants see data more than once or have to complete the same tasks more than once, this will affect their behaviors and opinions. In most cases, it can be avoided by using data and tasks that are not literally the same but similar with regard to the characteristics that matter. For example, in a study on grammatical factors that affect text difficulty, Leroy et al. [4, 5] compared a complex and easy version of text. The task was to answer questions posed about the text. Enormous differences in reading skills, medical background knowledge and reasoning skills could affect the study outcomes so a within-subjects design was preferred. Naturally, showing two versions, an easy and difficult version, of the same text would lead to a second look bias. It was therefore necessary to use two texts on different topics but with similar grammar characteristics.

Other Countermeasures

Sampling bias is the result of a nonrandom sample of participants or artifacts from the population. To counter sampling bias as much as possible, the researcher should use good sampling strategies. In short, this means that the researcher should use strategies such as trying to reach out to the entire relevant population in an interesting and understandable manner, making participation convenient, clearly showing the relevance and practical importance of participation and indicating that it is not abnormal to volunteer. However, sampling bias is difficult to counter. Therefore it is useful to compare the sample characteristics to the population characteristics. This will help put the conclusions in context. Such a comparison will provide an indication of how representative the sample was. Chapter 16 discusses how to check for such nonrandom samples.

The Hawthorne effect is commonly understood to mean a change in behaviors due to the effect of being monitored. A possible counter to this effect is to ensure that a good placebo condition is in effect that allows for similar measuring or monitoring without providing the treatment. For example, Smith et al. [6] conducted a study using a telemedicine intervention to improve sleep apnea patients' adherence to their prescribed treatment. The common and effective treatment for sleep apnea is continuous positive airway pressure. Unfortunately, adherence to the treatment is often low. The researchers worked with sleep apnea patients who had shown low adherence to the treatment and compared two telemedicine interventions that involved observing patients using their equipment. The treatment consisted of emphasizing the importance of adhering to the treatment while the placebo emphasized the important of taking vitamins. Both conditions applied the same type of telemedicine-based monitoring. The researchers found a significant effect of the treatment. Because they used a placebo condition involving the same monitoring and measurements, the effect could not be attributed to the novelty of the treatment or the act of being observed.

Beware of Overreacting

It is unnecessary to turn all nuisance variables into independent variables. Some might argue that since a nuisance variable has to be controlled to reduce its influence, it may as well be treated as an independent variable. However, nuisance variables are not independent variables. Independent variables are those that the developer or researcher is interested in: the variables that have a scientific or business interest behind them. Nuisance variables are not the main interest of the study. Including them as independent variables would increase the scope of the study, would require additional hypotheses and statistical testing, and would make the study more time consuming and expensive to conduct.

Naturally, variables may be considered nuisance variables in one study but independent variables in another. For example, assume a new information system for mobile devices to support weight loss. The new software is intended to be used for taking pictures of food, recognizing the items on the pictures and providing nutritional information. Since the software product is intended to be useful for and sold to both men and women, gender is a nuisance variable and should be controlled in the study. This could be done by ensuring that each experimental condition has an equal number of men and women. However, assume another information system where motivational text messages are sent under the assumption that men and women are motivated differently and will react differently to messages. In this case, the study should treat gender as an independent variable and measure the effect on men and women separately.

Bias is an important effect to counter. Countering bias does not need to be expensive or require many resources but careful design will be essential. However, the payoff of having a much better designed and controlled study will be substantial.

References

1. Leroy G, Leo GD, Fryer J (2007) An online community for teachers to support, observe, collect and evaluate assisted communication with children with autistic spectrum disorders who use smartphones as communication devices. Paper presented at the Workshop on intelligent systems for assisted cognition, Rochester, New York, 12–13 October 2007
2. Pouwer F, Snoek FJ, van der Ploeg HM, Heine RJ, Brand AN (1998) A comparison of the standard and the computerized versions of the well-being questionnaire (WBQ) and the diabetes treatment satisfaction questionnaire (DTSQ). Qual Life Res 7:33–38

3. Leroy G, Lally AM, Chen H (2003) The use of dynamic contexts to improve casual internet searching. ACM T Inform Syst 21(3):229–253
4. Leroy G, Helmreich S, Cowie J (2010) The influence of text characteristics on perceived and actual difficulty of health information. Int J Med Inform 79(6):438–449
5. Leroy G, Helmreich S, Cowie JR (2010) The effects of linguistic features and evaluation perspective on perceived difficulty of medical text. In: Hawaii international conference on system sciences (HICSS), Kauai, 5–8 January 2010
6. Smith CE, Dauz ER, Clements F, Puno FN, Cook D, Doolittle G, Leeds W (2006) Telehealth services to improve nonadherence: a placebo-controlled study. Telemed J E Health 12(3):289–296

Avoid Missing the Effect

14

Chapter Summary

Given the amount of time, money and effort that is spent on developing new algorithms and information systems, surprisingly little time is used to teach how to conduct a valuable evaluation. When evaluation is discussed, the focus is often on avoiding Type I errors, where a nonexistent effect is incorrectly accepted as existing. In contrast, this chapter focuses on Type II errors, where an existing effect is missed.

Type II errors often receive less attention even though, especially in medicine, making such errors may affect people's quality of life. When a new information system is built, it is intended to improve an existing medical problem. Missing an existing effect wastes time and effort of one group and may incorrectly put others off the trail, thereby stopping further research and development of a potentially promising approach. With good experimental design, the chances of this can be minimized. To avoid missing an effect, the difference between means of experimental conditions should be sufficiently large. The within-group variation should be relatively small so that the difference between groups is larger than that within groups. And a large enough number of observations should be made in each experimental condition, especially with smaller effect sizes.

Problems with Within- and Between-Group Variation

To describe the problems discussed in this section, a frequency distribution of scores is used as is shown in Fig. 14.1. Such a distribution is commonly used to show data and the characteristics of populations and samples (see also Chap. 3). The x-axis depicts the scores on the dependent variable. These are the measurements taken during an experiment. For example, in Fig. 14.1 there are three scores, $x1$, $x2$ and $x3$, shown for the dependent variable. On the y-axis are the frequencies of these scores. For example, $freq(x1)$ indicates how frequently score $x1$ was found in the sample. In this example, the score $x1$ is the most commonly found score. Scores $x2$ and $x3$ are

G. Leroy, *Designing User Studies in Informatics*, Health Informatics,
DOI 10.1007/978-0-85729-622-1_14, © Springer-Verlag London Limited 2011

Fig. 14.1 Frequency distribution

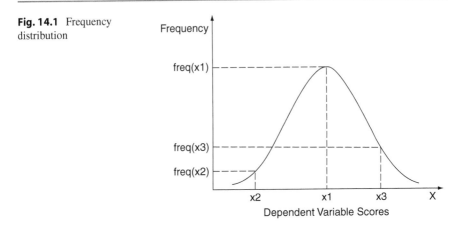

found less frequently. With many type of metrics, the frequency distribution will assume a bell shape. The bulk of the scores are centered on a central value, *x1* in the example, which is the mean score. The tails on both sides of the curve depict the extreme scores. This bell curve shows how the majority of scores are close together and how there are increasingly fewer extreme scores. For example, there are fewer people who scored *x3* than *x1*, as can be read from the distribution where *freq(x3)* is lower than *freq(x1)*. In this example, *x2* is even more extreme and *freq(x2)* is smaller than *freq(x3)*.

Figure 14.1 shows one curve representing one sample or population. When there are multiple experimental conditions, it is expected that the samples of each condition show different characteristics and so represent different populations. This would be evident from two distributions that each have a different mean and surrounding bell curve representing the frequency of scores. For example, in an experiment on learning, one sample may show improved results compared to the control condition. However, when the treatment is ineffective, only one bell curve will be observed. This chapter uses the bell curve representation to demonstrate common errors in experimental design and how to avoid them.

Figure 14.2 shows the results of a fictitious experiment with one independent variable that has two conditions. The figure is used to demonstrate a progressively improved experimental design that takes care of avoiding too little between-group variation and too much within-group variation. The intent of the researchers is to compare two conditions: Condition 1 and Condition 2. On the x-axis are the scores for the dependent variable for each condition. The y-axis shows the frequency of each score. Each curve represents one condition of the independent variable. The curve labeled Condition 1 shows the distribution of scores for the first condition of the independent variable and the curve labeled Condition 2 illustrates the second condition. Intuitively, think about the frequency (y-axis) as how representative a score is or how likely it is for a person with that score to belong to that condition. Since each curve belongs to a sample, two different curves can be seen as representative of two different populations when the statistical analysis indicates that these curves represent statistically different samples.

The example experiment evaluates fictitious new voice recognition software for dictating medical records. The software can be used out-of-the-box by English speakers and can recognize either a British or American accent. The software also provides the user the option to train it. The developers decide to evaluate the software in an experiment. Their first choice is to test the software with its out-of-the-box version as Condition 1 and compare it with Condition 2 where users train it for 15 min. For this example, assume that training the software leads to better outcomes. A variety of potential users, such as nurses, doctors and medical students, are randomly assigned to one of the two conditions. The users are recruited from a British university hospital and have a variety of backgrounds. In addition to British students, there are visiting scholars from the United States, Asia, Africa and Europe.

Too Little Between-Groups Variation

Figure 14.2a demonstrates how the means of the two experimental conditions are very close together. In such a situation, an existing effect may not be detected because there is not enough between-groups variation to lead to a statistically significant effect. Consider the observation o, which is one example score achieved by study participants. The score o is achieved by many people in Condition 1. It is high on the curve indicating the frequency of that score was high. But there are also many people in Condition 2 who achieved this same score as can be seen from the curve for Condition 2. The two frequencies *freq1(o)* and *freq2(o)* are close together. This example score shows how one score could very likely belong to Condition 1 but almost as likely to Condition 2. This is the case for many scores in Fig. 14.2a. There is much overlap between the curves which means that there are many scores that are fairly typical for both samples.

It is unclear from a result such as the one shown in Fig. 14.2a whether the two samples are representative of one population, which would be the case when the treatment has no effect, or whether the two samples are representative of two populations, which would be the case if there was a significant difference between treatments. The overlap between conditions will make it difficult to distinguish between them statistically. By using a better design and better sampling procedures, it is possible to see curves that are further apart representing conditions that are different.

For the given example of voice recognition software, there are several possible reasons why an existing effect was not detected. For example, the training time was very short and so the effect may have been very small. By using a longer training time, the effect would have been stronger and the means of the curves further apart. Alternatively, a third condition could have been added to the experiment with this longer training period. The outcome of such different conditions also would provide valuated information for the business' marketing approach. Some buyers would not train the software at all and it is important to know what kind of performance they can expect. Others will be willing to spend some time, so knowing how much time people would be willing to spend (a survey can help here) would be a good second condition. Finally, testing what the best possible performance would be can be done with intense and long training for a third condition.

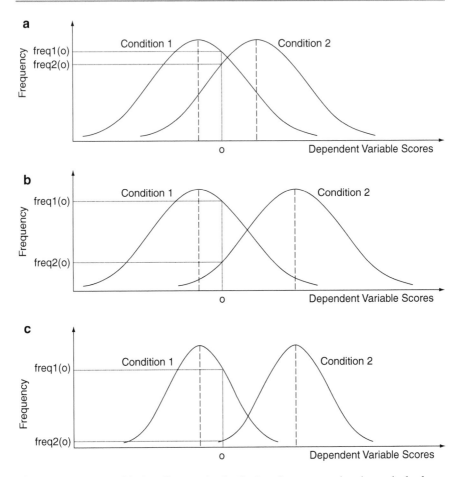

Fig. 14.2 Illustration of design effects on the distribution of scores: **a–c** show increasingly clearer effects

Figure 14.2b shows an improvement compared to Fig. 14.2a. It demonstrates the impact of having means that are further apart. In the given example, this could result from using more training time. Compared to Fig. 14.2a, the likelihood of a statistically significant difference in means being between conditions is better. Under the new conditions, the observation *o* is a common score in Condition 1 but not in Condition 2. The frequencies *freq1(o)* and *freq2(o)* are very different from each other in Fig. 14.2b.

Too Much Within-Groups Variation

Although Fig. 14.2b shows improvement, it also demonstrates the continued problem caused by too much variation of scores within each experimental group. To find the significant effect, the variation between the groups has to be higher than the variation within the groups (see discussion on ANOVA in Chap. 3). The curves in Fig. 14.2b are broad and there is much overlap between them. This overlap represents that part of each sample that could belong to either of the two conditions. Intuitively, narrower curves make it easier to see that the populations represented by the two samples are different. The researcher should consider controlling nuisance variables by using a blocked design to control one nuisance variable (see Chap. 5) or a Latin Square design to control multiple nuisance variables (see Chap. 6) to reduce unnecessary variation.

Narrowing the curves can be done by controlling bias and nuisance effects. For example, when designing an experiment, volunteers are randomly assigned to the experimental conditions. This does not mean that anybody should be qualified or be considered a representative participant. When participants share the same characteristics that affect the outcome, the variation in each group will be smaller. Inclusion and exclusion criteria are therefore an important aspect of the design. They should not be too narrow, since then the results cannot be generalized; however, they should not be too broad since then the participants will widely vary and there is an increased risk of higher variation in the group. For the given example, even with eligible participants the differences in native language between participants will lead to very different scores. Non-native English speakers have an accent which will affect the training process of voice recognition software. If many different accents are present in the sample, this will increase the variability. Other factors also may have contributed. For example, if participants brought their own texts for training, a wide variety of materials will be used. Software developed for medical health record dictation can be expected to perform differently with medical texts, compared to literature or poetry.

In addition to using careful sampling, other nuisance variables that can cause variation in scores may be related to the environment. When the environment matters and it differs for participants, it will add more variation to the scores. This variation is unrelated to the experimental treatment and should be controlled. For example, the example study may have been conducted in a university laboratory close to classrooms or an office close to the company's cafeteria. Even though all participants of Condition 2 trained the voice recognition software for the prescribed amount of time, the environment in which this took place changed between subjects. It may have been quiet for some subjects but noisy for others, for example, between classes or during the lunch break. Noise may have affected the speech recognition training and the resulting variation in scores therefore was much higher.

Figure 14.2c demonstrates the effect of lowering the variation in scores in each group. The result is that observed scores center more closely around the mean and there are fewer extremes. It is clear that there is little overlap between the curves. And even though the means in Fig. 14.2c are the same as in Fig. 14.2b, the differences between the two samples are much more pronounced. For example, the observation o in this version of the experiment is very likely to occur under Condition 1 but very unlikely to occur under Condition 2. Controlling nuisance variables will help decrease the variation of scores in each group.

Problems with Sample Size or Statistics

In addition to designing appropriate levels of the independent variables and controlling nuisance variables, having ample participants in each experimental condition of the study will improve the power of the study. Enough participants

Table 14.1 Number of subjects with between-subjects design

		IV 1:Training time		
		None	15 min	60 min
IV 2: Software used	Existing software	n1–n30	n31–n60	n61–n90
	New software	n91–n120	n121–n150	n151–n180

Table 14.2 Number of subjects with within-subjects design

		IV 1:Training time		
		None	15 min	60 min
IV 2: Software used	Existing software	n1–n30	n1–n30	n1–n30
	New software	n1–n30	n1–n30	n1–n30

are needed to show a statistically significant difference between conditions. The commonly used rule of thumb states that 30 participants are needed. It is important to keep in mind that this means that *30 observations* are suggested *per experimental condition*. The actual and total number of participants needed differs depending on the design principles used and the number of conditions for each independent variable. Keep in mind that the number 30 is a rule of thumb and that with weak effects more subjects will be needed, while with strong effects fewer subjects will be needed to show a statistically significant difference between experimental conditions.

Table 14.1 shows an example of a study with two independent variables that follows a between-subjects design. Each study subject is assigned to one experimental condition. If 30 observations are needed in each experimental condition there would be 180 subjects required: 6 groups of 30 participants.

Table 14.2 shows the same experiment but follows a within-subjects approach. In this example, only one group of 30 subjects is recruited and each subject participates in all experimental conditions. When people participate in such an experimental design, the order of conditions usually should be randomized for each subject. When the subjects are artifacts, randomization will not matter. However, in this example, because the difference between conditions for the first independent variable (training time) is time spent, the order of conditions should be retained and measurements should be taken before training, after 15 min of training and after 60 min of training. The order of the second independent variable (software) should be randomized: half of the subjects should first receive the existing software and the other half should first receive the new software. In this case, 30 subjects need to be recruited.

Several combinations of the between- and within-subjects principle are possible and can be applied to avoid bias or practical obstacles in conducting the experiment. It can be expected, for example, that training two types of voice recognition software during one experiment takes too much time for a person. The experimental design could be adjusted so that the first independent variable (training time) remains a within-subject variable, while the second independent variable (software) is treated as a between-subject variable. In this case, 60 subjects need to be recruited, as is shown in Table 14.3.

Table 14.3 Number of subjects with between- and within-subjects mixed design

		IV 1:Training time		
		None	15 min	60 min
IV 2: Software used	Existing software	n1–n30	n1–n30	n1–n30
	New software	n31–n60	n31–n60	n31–n60

Depending on the statistic used, there are a few more restrictions that need to be taken into account. When the t-test is used, it is important to have an equal number of participants (as equal as possible) in each condition. If the numbers of participants are not equal, an adjusted t-test will need to be conducted (see Chap. 3). See Rosenthal and Rosnow [1] (Chap. 15) for an overview of the effects on t when there are unequal numbers of participants in the different conditions of the experiment. For an overview of the Cell Means Model, an adjustment to the classical ANOVA approach, and how this can be adjusted to deal with unequal n and even empty cells in the design when conducting ANOVA, see Kirk [2] (Chaps. 9 and 10).

Increasing Power

The power of an experiment was discussed in Chap. 3 and is defined as in Eq. 14.1 where β is the probability of making a Type II Error. The power of an experiment depends on the independent variable's conditions, the dependent variable, the number of subjects who participate, the strength of the effect and the statistic used.

$$Power = 1 - \beta \qquad (14.1)$$

Power analysis can be done before and after a study. When power analysis is done before the start of an experiment, it can be used to calculate the sample size that would be needed to reach an alpha of a certain size, for example, .05 or .01. At this time, the most appropriate statistic can also be chosen. For example, when there is, in reality, a difference between means as hypothesized, a one-tailed t-test hypothesizing the correct direction will have more power than a two-tailed t-test. In addition, specifying the comparisons between conditions to be done in advance based on hypotheses also will result in a more powerful study since conducting multiple post hoc comparisons will require a Bonferonni adjustment (Chap. 8).

Depending on how strong the effect is, a different number of observations will be needed to detect a difference statistically. With smaller effects, more participants are needed. The number of participants needed can be calculated using the *effect-size index*. For example, when working with a t-test, the index is referred to by d, for an F-test by f and with χ^2 a w is used. An overview of the number of observations needed to detect small, medium or large effects at different alpha levels, for example, at .05 or .01, can be found in Cohen [3] and Rosenthal and Rosnow [1]. The actual numbers that indicate small, medium or large effects differ and also can be found in these sources.

When power analysis is done after the study has been completed, it is generally done to find out why no significant effect was detected. It is important to know whether the study did not have sufficient power or whether there was sufficient power but no effect. When the study did not have enough power, the existence of the effect has not been shown but it has not been rejected either. When a study had sufficient power and no effect was detected, this most likely means that there was no effect of the independent variable (given the study was well designed).

Thinking carefully about the conditions of an experiment will help increase the chances that an existing effect will be discovered. However, sometimes it takes more than having enough subjects or a well defined independent variable. The next chapter discusses how to avoid missing an effect when multiple variables or conditions are at play.

References

1. Rosenthal R, Rosnow RL (1991) Essentials of behavioral research: methods and data analysis. McGraw-Hill, Boston
2. Kirk RE (1995) Experimental design: procedures for the behavioral sciences, 3rd edn. Brooks/Cole Publishing Company, Pacific Grove
3. Cohen J (1988) Statistical power analysis for the behavioral sciences, 2nd edn. L. Erlbaum Associates, Hillsdale

Avoid Missing Variables or Conditions

15

Chapter Summary

This chapter continues the discussion of errors that can be avoided so that the outcome of the user study is maximized. While the previous chapter focused on the existing variables and how they can be optimized without changing the design of the study, this chapter demonstrates how an inferior study design and inappropriate analysis can lead to erroneous conclusions. First, the effects of missing an independent variable are explained by demonstrating how a missed interaction can lead to effects being cancelled out. Second, missing an important condition may also result in no effect being found at all. Finally, using ANOVA and its omnibus F-test may also lead to missing effects when the arrangement of conditions is important, for example, when the conditions represent a linear trend.

Missing an Important Variable

When developing an information system, it is not always clear which user or environmental characteristics will affect the use of the system. Ideally, the information system is useful to as many people as possible and provides an advantage over the previous situation. The user study is conducted to verify such positive impact. Unfortunately, some information systems are not as generally effective as intended, and different outcomes may be found for different people, tasks, situations or environments. When this is the case, the outcome of a user study may be unclear and any positive effects may be disguised. It is then possible that advantages of the new system are completely missed because another source of variance obscured the results. The source of variance may have been a variable that was important but ignored. Its interaction with the experimental variable was missed. Ideally, this is discovered during the pilot study so that the design of the full study can be adjusted. Alternatively, if the effect was not suspected and discovered until after the study was completed, a post hoc analysis may still be a valuable approach to estimating the effect.

G. Leroy, *Designing User Studies in Informatics*, Health Informatics,
DOI 10.1007/978-0-85729-622-1_15, © Springer-Verlag London Limited 2011

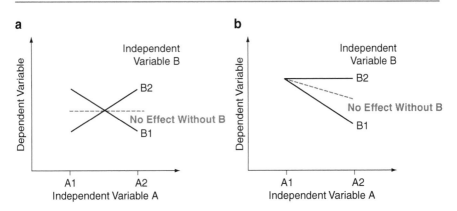

Fig. 15.1 Examples of missed interaction effects

Figure 15.1a shows an idealized demonstration of this problem. Independent Variable A represents the comparison between an old (Condition 1) and new (Condition 2) information system. The figure demonstrates how the information system is used very differently or leads to very different outcomes when Independent Variable B is taken into account. If Variable B were not included in this study, no difference would have been found between the two conditions (represented by the dotted line). The researchers would conclude that there was no significant difference between using the old system and the new one. The effect of the information system is masked because the interaction effect between the two independent variables is missed. The outcome differs for the old compared to the new information system – in this case the results diverge – depending on the condition of Variable B.

For example, Leroy and Miller [1] worked on visualizing the structure of health text to improve document comprehension. Although the system was intended to be helpful to all readers of the text, the system was only effective for those readers who had low health literacy. Analyzing the results for all user data as one group would not have shown any significant effect of the system. However, because users were grouped according to their health literacy, a clear effect was found. People with low health literacy interacted differently with the information system compared to those with high health literacy: they relied much more on the information system to help them provide answers to the questions.

Figure 15.1b shows another example of a missed effect. In this case, the problem is due to the information system being less generic than hoped and having an effect only for a subset of situations or users. If Variable B were not included in the study, the results would have shown a slight, but most probably insignificant, difference between the two conditions of Variable A. Because the effect exists only for a sub-group of the users, it does not surface when all results are combined. The effect of the information system in one group is overcome by the lack of differences between the other observations.

These conditions also demonstrate the usefulness of pilot studies. They are a good approach to discovering potentially important variables so that they can be taken into account for the full study. However, if this problem is discovered after conducting the full study and the existence of such a missed variable is suspected, dividing the subjects afterward into groups may still be very useful. For example, Leroy et al. [2] showed evidence that people's expertise using search engines impacted their interaction with different search engine algorithms. The overall goal of the study was to test search engine algorithms that were developed to improve the queries formed by users and thereby help them search the web. Using a within-subjects design, 5 search algorithms were compared using a search task that required the subjects to find answers to difficult questions. Both precision and recall were calculated but showed very little difference between the conditions. However, the subjects were also divided into three groups based on their overall achievement in answering the questions. When the results were evaluated per group, it was clear that the three groups interacted differently with the algorithms. One algorithm was particularly helpful to low achievers but did not help the high and middle achiever groups.

Although a post hoc discovery is not nearly as powerful as controlling the effect, checking for a missed variable is an interesting addition to the results and can help explain the lack of an effect. Unfortunately, in many cases the post hoc constructed groups are unbalanced and the statistical analysis is therefore complicated. In the worst case, the researchers may have to rely solely on a visual inspection of the results. Moreover, even when there are sufficient subjects to test this missing variable post hoc, the subjects were not randomly assigned to the conditions and so the requirements for an experiment are not met. The study may need to be considered a quasi-experiment.

Missing an Important Condition

When conducting studies, experience and knowledge of the subject matter is important and will result in better designed experiments and more relevant conclusions. This is especially the case when different levels of an independent variable need to be evaluated. Good knowledge and some intuition of the optimal conditions for an information system will help ensure that important conditions are not missing from the experiment.

Figure 15.2 is an idealized representation that shows how failing to test a condition may lead a researcher to conclude that there is no effect. It shows the results of an experiment in which two conditions, Condition 1 and Condition 2, show no difference in scores. If these were the only two conditions tested, the researcher would have concluded that the independent variable had no effect: the average scores for Condition 1 and Condition 2 are the same. However, it is possible that both conditions were too extreme. This may happen when the independent variable is a continuous variable. For example, with informatics-based persuasion approaches encouraging people to lead a healthier lifestyle, researchers may find that sending one persuasive message may not be effective, while sending many persuasive messages, such as every hour, may similarly be ineffective. In the former case there is not enough persuasion interaction, and in the latter there is too much and subjects get annoyed. In such situations, the optimal condition has been missed.

Fig. 15.2 Illustration of a missing condition

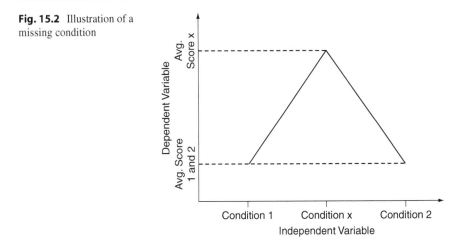

When the different conditions for an independent variable are chosen, it is not always clear what optimum levels need to be tested. In studies where two conditions are compared, for example, a low and high level of the independent variable, much depends on the exact levels that are being chosen. Complicating matters is that the researcher may have several options from which to choose. In other cases, where an existing situation with an old or no information system is compared with a new information system, the options will be more limited.

Missing Other Effects

While effects may be missed because a condition or variable is not included in an experiment, the effect may also be missed when the conditions are not sufficiently different for an ANOVA to detect. An ANOVA is the obvious choice to conduct an analysis in experiments where there are multiple conditions for at least one independent variable. However, it may miss effects because it does not take the arrangements of the conditions into account. For example, when different conditions represent a linear increase in the amount of therapy, this is not tested with an ANOVA. It is important to keep in mind that an ANOVA uses an omnibus F-test. It evaluates whether there are any differences between the conditions that are significant. For example, even if the outcome correlates with the increased levels of treatment, this will not necessarily be detected as a significant effect by an ANOVA.

Choosing conditions that differ widely is not always possible. For example, Leroy et al. found that the number of function words in a text, such as pronouns or auxiliaries, affects the perceived difficulty of a text [3–6]. In a pilot study [6], five versions of a sentence were compared. The sentences differed only in the number of function words that were used. Since all sentences needed to be grammatically correct, there was a limit on the number of function words that could be added. As a result, the difference between experimental conditions also was limited. In the pilot study,

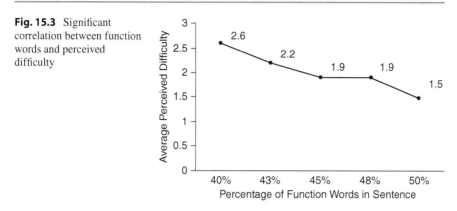

Fig. 15.3 Significant correlation between function words and perceived difficulty

10 subjects evaluated each sentence and indicated on a Likert scale (with a 1–4 range) how difficult to read they considered the sentences to be. A score of 1 indicated an easy sentence and a score of 4 indicated a difficult sentence. Figure 15.3 shows that there was a negative correlation between the number of function words and the difficulty ratings ($r = -0.960$, $p < .01$): having fewer functions words was correlated with higher perceived difficulty. However, a repeated measures ANOVA did not show a significant main effect ($p=.142$). Naturally, it is possible that working with more subjects for this study would have made the F-test significant. However, this is not guaranteed and would have depended on the variability of scores in each condition.

The researcher should carefully consider the goal of the study and choose the appropriate analysis. A standard ANOVA is useful to evaluate whether there are significant differences between conditions. However, this analysis does not take linear or other relationships between the conditions of the independent variable into account. A correlation analysis can be more appropriate or can be conducted in addition to the ANOVA. Alternatively, the researcher can also test with linear contrasts for relationships such as the one demonstrated in the example explained above. Testing for a linear relationship did yield a significant result for the percentage of function words in a sentence ($p =.012$).

References

1. Leroy G, Miller T (2010) Perils of providing visual health information overviews for consumers with low health literacy or high stress. J Am Med Inform Assoc 17:220–223. doi:doi:10.1136/jamia.2009.002717
2. Leroy G, Lally AM, Chen H (2003) The use of dynamic contexts to improve casual internet searching. ACM T Inform Syst 21(3):229–253
3. Leroy G (2008) Improving health literacy with information technology. In: Wickramasinghe N (ed) Encyclopaedia of healthcare information systems. Idea Group Inc, Hershey
4. Leroy G, Helmreich S, Cowie J (2010) The influence of text characteristics on perceived and actual difficulty of health information. Int J Med Inform 79(6):438–449

5. Leroy G, Helmreich S, Cowie JR (2010) The effects of linguistic features and evaluation perspective on perceived difficulty of medical text. In: Hawaii international conference on system sciences (HICSS), Kauai, 5–8 January 2010
6. Leroy G, Helmreich S, Cowie JR, Miller T, Zheng W (2008) Evaluating online health information: beyond readability formulas. In: AMIA, Washington DC, 8–12 November 2008

Other Errors to Avoid

16

Chapter Summary

This chapter continues the discussion of errors that can be avoided without requiring an extraordinary amount of time or resources but that would, when not avoided, seriously weaken the study design. The errors discussed in this chapter are typically made when researchers want to speed up the evaluation process by spending less time on applied tasks such as collecting test data or installing comparison systems. These errors are made when researchers reuse test data during the evaluation or when they use a demo or default version of comparison systems. Both cases result in an unfair comparison of the new system with another: the first because the system has been tuned to the test data and will perform unusually well, and the second because the comparison system is used in a substandard version and will perform unusually poorly. Then, two other types of errors are discussed, one when no time is spent verifying that the randomization of subjects was successful, and lastly when carelessly constructed Likert scales are used.

Confusing Development and Evaluation

Both complete information systems and individual algorithms benefit from multiple evaluations. A system will be much more stable, robust and effective when it and its algorithms are frequently tested. The software development process is a step-wise process during which the algorithms become increasingly more complete and complex. With more complete algorithms, more realistic data can be used for testing. When algorithms are combined, increasingly larger portions of the information system can be evaluated. Most software development life cycles are not linear processes but require cycles of development and testing. It is tempting to use the test data from early cycles in the formal evaluations. However, this does not provide a realistic picture of the capabilities of the final system.

It is essential that the development and evaluation activities are clearly separated regardless of when during the software development life cycle the evaluation takes

G. Leroy, *Designing User Studies in Informatics*, Health Informatics,
DOI 10.1007/978-0-85729-622-1_16, © Springer-Verlag London Limited 2011

place. This is to ensure that the evaluation is trustworthy and that it provides useful information for external evaluators and for further improvement of the system. Frequently, developers violate these principles and data or tasks that were used for testing are reused in the user studies. Since the data was used to develop and fine-tune the system, conclusions from an evaluation using this data would be limited to that particular dataset while the performance with new data or tasks remains unknown.

User studies in medical informatics are commonly classified as formative or summative evaluations [1, 2] (see also Chap. 1). A formative evaluation is done while the system or algorithm is still being developed. A summative evaluation is the final evaluation, done at the point in time when there will be no more changes. In this case, the information system is typically tested in its intended environment. Both types of evaluation should be performed separately from the development activities. The three phases of testing are described below to clearly distinguish them from each other.

Testing During Development

Researchers and developers working on an information system or algorithm should gather a dataset that is representative of the data that will be used by the final system. Initially this dataset can be taken from simulated data, but increasingly real examples will be required. The developer selects the data that is relevant to test a portion of the algorithm or system. Simple, cleansed data without exceptions or special cases is usually preferred at this stage since the basic functionality has to be demonstrated first. During the development process, problems are discovered in response to such data processing. These problems are fixed, and the same and new data examples are then used to continue testing. Ideally, the next round of development is started when a stable system state has been reached. The data used for testing is chosen with increasing complexity. When human interaction is required (for example, people interacting with the system's interface or evaluating its output) such testing will be conducted in the same fashion as with other types of data.

The testing result in this phase is unsuitable for publication in commercial or academic, peer-reviewed outlets. The results are in most cases not representative, often biased and seldom randomly selected. Furthermore, during ad hoc testing, there is significant bias at play. The data is carefully selected to test functionality; it does not represent the intended range of tasks, users or environment.

Once a stable state has been reached, the next stage can be a study to formatively evaluate the system. Ideally, this study is designed with input from developers so that it serves their further development activities.

Formative Evaluation

A formative evaluation, also called a constructive evaluation, is conducted during the design process before the information system is finalized (see also Chap. 1). These evaluations are very suitable for testing individual algorithms or standalone components such as, for example, a user interface. The evaluation is executed before the product has been finalized and is therefore intended to be helpful in providing direction for future development.

The goal of formative evaluations is to help pinpoint problems and potential areas for improvement and to demonstrate the performance of the systems. It fits very well with iterative software development processes. By conducting these evaluations in a proper manner, the study will have internal validity and the results can be used to inform future development. Depending on the focus of the study, the external validity may be low. For example, when testing an individual algorithm, it will be difficult to generalize this evaluation to broad, realistic conditions. However, the broader the dataset, tasks and user interactions that are included in the study and, moreover, the more these resemble the intended usage of the system, the higher the external validity will be.

The focus of a formative evaluation can be a comparison with another existing system or it can consist of a comparison with another baseline, such as no system, or different versions of the new system. The latter case occurs because early on there may be no comparative system available or it is more important to choose between different options for the new system.

For a formative evaluation to be valuable, the design considerations discussed in this book need be taken into account. For example, experimenter bias needs to be avoided by having someone other than the designer or developer conduct the study. In addition, a data bias needs to be avoided by ensuring that the dataset used is different from that used during earlier development and testing. The existing dataset provides an unfair and unrealistic advantage to the new system. In addition, representative users, different from the developers, are also of utmost importance. Developers and designers are close to their projects; they know the ins and outs of the system. Bringing in new, representative users is required and will be informative for the developers. These users will have their own mental model and expectations of how the system should function which will be different from those of the developers.

Sometimes formative evaluations are used solely to improve future versions of the system and there is no intention or interest to publish the results. In that case, there may also be no interest in finding statistically different results between different versions. If the focus is on discovering as many potential problems as possible, fewer subjects are needed to conduct the study since a large portion of problems can be captured with a small number of subjects. In addition, when the results of the evaluation will only be used for product improvement, the study does not qualify as being research and when the risk to participants is minimal, no IRB review is necessary.

Summative Evaluation

A summative evaluation is conducted when all components have been developed and integrated and the development activities have been completed (see also Chap. 1). Ideally, the information system is placed in its intended environment for this evaluation. Two types of summative evaluation are used: short term and longitudinal evaluations. Either or both types can be conducted for an information system. Ideally, the results of both will point in the same direction. In practice, better results may be found with longitudinal evaluations when more time has passed by and users have become more practiced and comfortable using the new system.

A comparison with an existing situation or system is often done with a short term study. Representative users are randomly assigned to the new system or the baseline system. Naturally, the study is conducted using representative data. Since a summative evaluation is the final evaluation, the system is tested in its intended, often final, setting. The special considerations discussed in Chap. 1 should be reviewed: until a system used in a medical setting has been proven to be superior compared to the existing system and has been shown to do no harm, special care and precautions are needed. This may complicate the study. For example, when a new information system is integrated in a clinical environment, is it difficult, sometimes impossible, to randomly assign the new system or the old system to study participants. Creative solutions can consist of using the new system as a shadow system that does not affect the actual outcomes or using both systems in parallel, ensuring that quality of care is not interrupted.

Substandard Baselines: Demos and Defaults

In many cases, a new algorithm or information system is developed because it is believed it can be better than an existing system. A user study is conducted to verify whether this is true. The study needs to be designed so that the new approach is compared to the existing one. However, the existing solution is not always readily available for the study or cannot always be easily acquired, integrated and installed. In such cases, it is tempting to use an easy-to-install demo version or default values because it is faster and more convenient in the short run. Unfortunately, that usually does not allow a valid comparison. This difficulty may arise with both individual algorithms and information systems.

When algorithms are being evaluated, it may be possible to compare the existing and new algorithms directly. When the existing algorithms are made available as a service, a comparison can be made by using them as such. In other cases, the details of the algorithms may have been published so that they can be developed in-house. If the comparison point is a complete information system, including it in the study may be complicated. The information system may need to be acquired, installed and integrated in an environment before it can be used, or it may require substantial optimization and fine-tuning before it can serve as a valid comparison point. In addition, if it is already used in a specific setting, the study designers should consider this place as the potential study site.

In many cases, a "light" or demo version of an existing system is readily available. It may seem the ideal solution for inclusion in a user study. However, the danger is that it may not be possible to sufficiently tune and optimize this system to have a valid comparison point. Moreover, many demo versions do not include the full functionality of the system or cannot be adjusted to a specific situation. Working with such a version is a mistake when it does not provide an honest comparison. Then the validity of conclusions is in doubt. Care should be taken that the existing systems and algorithms are included in the study as they were intended to be used.

A similar mistake is made when developers have access to existing systems but lack the knowledge or the time to prepare those systems. They may choose to use the system default settings when comparing to the new information system. For example, *k-means* is a clustering algorithm where the number of clusters is chosen in advance. Most software packages include a default setting, for example, the default is 2 in SPSS (Version 16.0 for Windows). This number of clusters will not be suitable for all tasks. When comparing a new clustering algorithm with the k-means algorithm, using this default setting may lead a researcher to conclude that k-means is unsuitable and that the new algorithm is better. However, using the default values leads to this conclusion. Similar to the use of a demo version, such a study has limited validity.

Both demo versions and default values often lead to invalid conclusions when they do not include the necessary functions for a comparison. No claims can be made about the superiority of the new system compared to the old. The baseline condition is not comparable to any realistic condition since it uses limited functionality or default settings that were not adapted to the situation, tasks or users.

Not Verifying Randomization

The randomization process to assign study participants or artifacts to experimental conditions was discussed in Part I. In short, subjects can be assigned to a randomly chosen condition when they sign up, or the participants' numbers can be randomly distributed to the different conditions before the start of the study. Alternatively, when subjects partake in all experimental conditions, the order of conditions should be randomized for each of them. Tables with random numbers are available from statistical manuals [3–6] or random number generators available from software products can be used to make the assignments.

By not randomizing the subjects or artifacts to the experimental conditions, much validity is lost and the conclusions cannot be generalized beyond the experiment. Therefore, researchers should verify that the randomization process was successful. To do this, they should collect the necessary data during the study. This data should capture the relevant descriptive characteristics of the subjects to verify the study sample is representative of the population and also that the study samples do not differ systematically between conditions. For example, age, education level, language and computer proficiency are characteristics often assumed to be the same in all experimental conditions. If one experimental group has much more computer experience or is much younger, this may affect the results. Similarly, if the study sample is much younger than the intended population, the results cannot be generalized to that population. Depending on the study and intended population, the characteristics that need to be measured and verified will differ.

Once the relevant data has been collected, a chi-square (χ^2) analysis needs to be conducted. This analysis was discussed in detail in Chap. 3. Chi-square analysis allows the researcher to compare expected and observed frequencies. For example, when equal participation is expected of men and women in each experimental condition, the analysis can be used to check whether there is a discrepancy between the observed and expected frequencies. The outcome of the analysis indicates whether the difference is statistically significant. To verify that the randomization process worked, the researcher should use chi-square analysis to show that there is no statistical difference between observed and expected frequencies for each variable that is relevant to the study and sample.

Using a random assignment process is not a guarantee that the subjects or artifacts are randomly distributed with regard to the characteristics that matter. Unforeseen circumstances or unknown events may play a role. In addition, random assignment is not always practically possible. For example, when the subjects are nurses on a ward, it will be nearly impossible to assign nurses on the same ward to different conditions. In this case, entire ward will be assigned to an experimental condition with all nurses working there. To have true randomization in such a case, each ward would have to be considered as one data point and sufficient wards would need to be found to participate. This is seldom feasible. In such cases, a quasi-experiment may be the best solution, keeping in mind that due to a lack of randomization, there may be systematic differences between subjects in different experimental conditions. This may lead to confounding variables or bias. Minimizing potential bias and confounding and measuring with additional data collection will yield the most valuable results.

Useless Likert Scales

Likert scaling is a type of *summative scaling* or *summated rating* [4] that is used as an *attitude scale* to measure subjects' feelings and opinions on a specific topic. Each statement in the scale is intended to measure an aspect of that general attitude and the subjects' responses are summed into a final score. Many examples of Likert scales relevant to the researcher's topic can be found in the literature and, if they are validated, researchers should consider reusing these existing scales. Likert scales are often used to complement objective evaluations or other types of data gathering methods. For example, in a study of a new physician order entry system, Van Doormaal et al. [7] used 5-point Likert scales in addition to open-ended questions for their semi-structured interview of physicians and nurses.

Likert scales consist of a statement followed by a 5- or 7-point scale indicating various levels of agreement. The statement is expressed so that it is easily classifiable as favorable or unfavorable. The answer scales indicate the degree of agreement or disagreement with the statement. A 5-point Likert scale will show the following choices: Strongly Agree, Agree, Neutral, Disagree, Strongly Disagree; a 7-point Likert scale shows a more fine-grained scale, such as: Strongly Agree, Agree, Somewhat Agree, Neutral, Somewhat Disagree, Disagree, Strongly

Disagree. There are some additional adjustments that can be made to this type of scale. For example, a "Not Applicable" option can be provided to allow subjects to indicate when an item is not relevant to them. Or, researchers can decide to use a Likert scale without the middle neutral statement resulting in a 4-point or 6-point Likert scale.

As Rosenthal [4] describes it, Likert scales are "among the most misused terms in behavioral science." In medical informatics as well as in information and computer science, the "Likert scale" also is used very casually to evaluate opinions about information systems. The ease with which surveys can be distributed, answered and scored using online and often free tools has most likely contributed to their overuse. Often little effort is expended in composing a scale. However, with basic insight into the process, a better and more efficient instrument can be developed for which the results can be better trusted to be unbiased and true. For example, Garamendi [8] showed how a thoughtful approach and evaluation of a survey will lead to a much better instrument. The group evaluated a Quality of Life survey to be used with myopic patients who undergo surgery to correct the problem. Their analysis showed how items can be unnecessary and unclear and how a much more concise and relevant survey can result from a well executed evaluation.

Providing a complete tutorial on how to compile and validate a good Likert scale is beyond the scope of this book. The researcher should consult relevant manuals, such as [9], to construct, test and analyze the scale. In short, this means that, after initial construction, the scale and its items need to be tested in a pilot study with the target population. Item analysis should then be conducted to select a subset of items that best represent the scale and that correlate with the total score. *Cronbach's alpha*, a coefficient of reliability, is often used to verify this consistency. Only a scale that is carefully constructed and verified can be accepted as valid and reliable. When an extensive construction process and analysis are not within the means of the researchers, there are several precautions that should be taken when constructing the scale. Evaluating this scale as part of a pilot study will help improve the survey and make the resulting data more useful, reliable and valid. Below are a few guidelines to keep in mind.

List the Items

The first step in constructing a Likert scale is to define what the attitude or opinion is that will be measured and to list the different aspects that need to be evaluated. The researchers should be systematic in this so that a complete picture is captured by the survey. In informatics, some common aspects to keep in mind are:
- All the different system components, such as the interface and even the help manuals,
- All the different qualitative aspects, such as the overall look and feel, perceived speed or the ease of learning,
- All required tasks and interactions with the system
- And the timescale of interest, such as past, current or future use.

One Statement per Item

With a Likert scale it is crucial to avoid double-barreled statements. When an item consists of two statements, easily recognized by a conjunction in the language, it will be unclear what is asked and what any answer means. For example, when an item contains the question whether a user likes component A *or* component B, these two components are confounded. It is unclear how a respondent should and will answer when he likes both or only one of the components. Similar questions will arise when an item contains whether the user likes component A *and* component B.

For example, a statement such as "The program helped me eat better and exercise more" contains two statements: one about eating and one about exercising. When respondents answer, it will not be clear whether they are answering that both were true or just one. It may be the intention of the researcher to check whether both were true, but many respondents will not read it as such or will be confused what to answer when they agree with only part of the statement. Even when respondents are systematic in how they answer such questions and use correct logic such as expected from truth tables, the researchers will not be able to verify this. It is much better to ensure there are no double-barreled statements. In the above example, the researchers should use two items: "The program helped me eat better" and "The program helped me exercise more."

Clear Language

The statements should be checked for grammar, spelling and style. Presenting a scale that looks professional will help ensure that respondents take it seriously. In addition to using correct language, it is essential that the vocabulary, grammar, tone and style of the statements are adjusted for the intended respondents. Respondents need to be able to understand the statements. For example, with low literacy populations, it will be essential to use easy-to-understand language. It is also essential that respondents and researchers assign the same meaning to terms. Therefore, slang should be avoided unless it is part of the respondents' language, and even then, the regular language alternatives should be included. Without such clear language, the internal validity of the survey will be very low since respondents will be answering items that represent different statements to different people.

Suitability

Especially with the option of using the Internet for data collection, it has become much easier to invite participants from different backgrounds, cultures and countries to answer the same survey. Whether the audience is broadly or narrowly defined, it remains extremely important to ensure that the items are suitable for the intended respondents to answer. This means that the language has to be appropriate as well as the tone and topics. For example, when working with children, it will be necessary to adjust the vocabulary so they can understand the questions.

The researcher should keep in mind that answering Likert scale items may be a Western approach to gathering opinions and not suitable for all. The need for consistency is not present in all cultures in this manner. This type of scale was developed in and for a Western culture preference of cognitive consistency; other cultures have been shown to be much more open to inconsistency [10]. Such Western ideas have led to items or data being disregarded when answers were considered inconsistent.

Length

The length of the statements needs to be tested to ensure they are not too long or it is likely they will not be read in their entirety. With such statements it is also easier to make mistakes such as using incorrect grammar or including double-barreled statements, and it is often more difficult for people to understand the statement.

In addition to the length of individual statements, it is essential that the list of statements, the entire survey, is not too long. Once a list becomes too long, participants may become bored or tired and this will affect their answers. With long surveys, there is also an increasing chance that participants will not complete the survey. A pilot study can help identify which items can be deleted. When two items measure the same attitude or feeling, one of them can be removed. When items do not correlate with the overall score they also can be removed since they measure something not relevant to the intended topic of the survey.

To help participants judge the length of a survey, it is helpful to show them their progress. For example, when the survey is online a progress bar can show how far along in the entire survey the participant is. This may help avoid participants quitting before completing the survey.

Consistency

The scale should have a consistent look. This can be accomplished by verifying that the scale options remain the same and in the same direction. Be especially careful when parts of the scale are added from a previous scale. Keeping the same direction in the answer options is crucial since most respondents will read the options only for the first few items. Then participants usually assume the same options are repeated. For example, if the direction of the options is switched, it will very likely go unnoticed and the evaluation will result in nonsense data. If the direction of the statements is switched to counter potential answering bias, for example, some respondents tend to answer 'to the right', then respondents should be made aware that they should read all options carefully.

It goes without saying that when the survey is presented online, it is essential that it is tested using different browsers, devices and screen sizes. This will help identify statements that are too long and verify that the progress bar shows progress correctly and, of utmost importance, that the data collection tools work.

In general, designing a user study should be done carefully to avoid common pitfalls and obstacles. Some well known problems were listed in the four chapters in this part. They do not require extraordinary resources, but when they can be avoided they will significantly improve the quality and outcomes of the study. With carefully designed user studies, the gains may be enormous. They include improvements in the current design, the future design, an evaluation of the system's potential, a first or in-depth interaction with potential customers, and ideally an improvement in the quality of life of many users.

References

1. Friedman CP, Wyatt JC (2000) Evaluation methods in medical informatics. Springer-Verlag, New York
2. Brender J (2006) Handbook of evaluation methods for health informatics (trans: Carlander L). Elsevier Inc, San Diego
3. Vaughan L (2001) Statistical methods for the information professional: a practical, painless approach to understanding, using, and interpreting statistics. Commercial statistics. Information Today, Inc, New Jersey
4. Rosenthal R, Rosnow RL (1991) Essentials of behavioral research: methods and data analysis. McGraw-Hill, Boston
5. Kirk RE (1995) Experimental design: procedures for the behavioral sciences, 3rd edn. Brooks/Cole Publishing Company, Pacific Grove
6. Kurtz NR (1999) Statistical analysis for the social sciences. Social sciences - statistical methods. Allyn & Bacon, Needham Heights
7. van Doormaal JE, Mol PGM, Zaal RJ, van den Bemt PMLA, Kosterink JGW, Vermeulen KM, Haaijer-Ruskamp FM (2010) Computerized physician order entry (CPOE) system: expectations and experiences of users. J Eval Clin Pract (Online). doi:10.1111/j.1365-2753.2009.01187.x
8. Garamendi E, Pesudovs K, Stevens MJ, Elliott DB (2006) The refractive status and vision profile: evaluation of psychometric properties and comparison of Rasch and summated Likert-scaling. Vis Res 46:1375–1383
9. Dunn-Rankin P, Knezek GA (2004) Scaling methods, 2nd edn. Lawrence Erlbaum Associates, Inc., Mahwah
10. Carr SC, Bishop DMG (1995) Attitude assessment in non-Western countries: critical modifications to Likert-scaling. Psychologia 39:55–59

Appendix: Cookbook for Designing User Studies in Informatics

Recipe 1: Evaluating Standalone Algorithms Using Artifacts

Recipe Summary

Figure A.1.1 shows an overview of the recipes discussed in this section. This recipe discusses the evaluation of an algorithm when there are no other suitable algorithms for comparison. The algorithm is assumed to process artifacts, i.e., man-made objects such as diagnostic images or medical records, and can be evaluated without interaction with the future users. The algorithm will be integrated and combined with other components into a complete information system in later phases in the system development life cycle. One independent variable will focus on the algorithm in comparison to a valid baseline. The evaluation demonstrated in this recipe can often be conducted by sampling representative artifacts from a set and using a within-subjects design.

Place in the Development Life Cycle and Example

Evaluating individual algorithms before they are integrated is a good practice and helps design stable software. Advanced software, whether in the medical field or not, relies on the combination of several algorithms to perform special tasks. For example, search engines rely on indexing and matching algorithms, while decision support systems rely on algorithms to combine and visualize information. It is advisable not to wait until the entire system has been developed before conducting an evaluation. In most cases, the evaluation of an individual algorithm helps establish expectations when there are no similar algorithms to compare against. This situation occurs when new approaches are made possible by advances in computer hardware or when an algorithm is applied in a new context – for example, when a visualization algorithm for geographical data is applied to medical data.

There are many benefits to testing algorithms early in the development process. With a systematic evaluation of each component, one surprise factor is eliminated.

G. Leroy, *Designing User Studies in Informatics*, Health Informatics,
DOI 10.1007/978-0-85729-622-1, © Springer-Verlag London Limited 2011

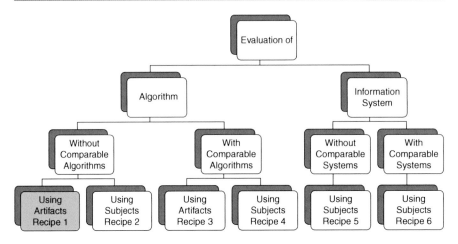

Fig. A.1.1 Standalone algorithm evaluation with artifacts

Problems are identified earlier and the causes of problems are easier to pinpoint. As a consequence, it will be much faster and cheaper to fix problems that are discovered. Although it could be argued that early testing may slow down the overall development cycle, that it costs extra money, or that it is too difficult, research has shown that problems should be caught as early as possible. The price tag associated with fixing problems becomes increasingly larger later in the process [1].

For this recipe, it is assumed there is an existing dataset that contains representative artifacts that can be used during the evaluation. For example, for a new prediction algorithm that uses information in medical records, the artifacts are the medical records. When this dataset is sufficiently large, several evaluations can be done. Each will fit in a development cycle and so the effectiveness of the algorithm can be enhanced.

Applied Example

In this chapter, the following fictitious example is used to illustrate individual steps.

A new algorithm has been developed that can distinguish between the seasonal flu and the H1N1 variant (swine flu). The seasonal flu often includes a range of symptoms such as fever, coughing, sore throat, runny/stuffy nose, headaches, body aches, chills and fatigue. Additional symptoms of the H1N1 flu are often, but not always, diarrhea and vomiting. A company has mined online blogs for complaints associated with both types of flu, as well as additional information related to time of infection, contact with others and general descriptive information such as age, gender and general health. This information was used to train a prediction algorithm. The novelty of the algorithm is that it uses only information that can be gained by speaking with a patient. As such, it can be used during a phone interview or online chat session and is thereby cheaper, faster and more effective in stopping the spread of the disease. The researchers in the company who developed this algorithm are interested in including the algorithm in a symptom checker for mobile devices.

Choose the Dataset

The dataset consists of those artifacts that the algorithm will process. Ideally, a large set of these artifacts is available or can be constructed. A subset of artifacts can be used during development testing, but it is essential that they are not reused in the evaluation phase as this does not allow for an honest evaluation. During the development phases, the algorithm is continuously improved based on errors discovered using specific artifacts. As a result, the algorithm has been tuned or, at a minimum, been adjusted sufficiently using these examples so that few or no further errors will be found. It would be an incorrect representation of the algorithm's capabilities to then use this data for evaluation.

If all artifacts are similar, randomly select examples for use during the development phase. However, in many projects there will be different groups of artifacts, for example, simple and complex artifacts, that need to be handled by the algorithm. In this case, choose examples from all groups for development and testing. These can be chosen by the developers for particular characteristics, such as the presence of certain symbols or extreme data ranges. For the evaluation discussed here, all groups should be represented. This can be accomplished with stratified random sampling from the artifacts. No artifacts should be reused from the development cycles.

The complete dataset used for evaluation should contain at least 30 artifacts for each experimental condition. This ensures that enough data points will be available for statistical testing. The rule of thumb is to have 30 data points in each experimental condition because at that point the Student's t-distribution approaches the normal distribution. In this recipe, where an existing algorithm is tested and compared against a baseline (defined below), a within-subjects or between-subjects approach can be used for the evaluation. In the first case, a minimum of 30 examples will be needed, in the latter 60 or more. Keep in mind that a study has more power to detect even small effects when there are more data points per condition. The statistical analysis discussed here requires equal sample sizes in the different experimental conditions.

Applied Example

The algorithm was developed after a biomedical researcher in the company had a key insight. During development, he questioned his family members and friends for their symptoms and doctor's diagnosis. He also collected online patient blogs and descriptions from websites which where transcribed into datasets. These examples were used to develop and test rules. The researcher felt the rules to be complete and wanted to conduct a formal evaluation. Luckily, his company is affiliated with a large university hospital that keeps electronic health records for all patients. It turns out there are 5,000 records of flu-related cases. In 2,000 cases, the records indicate H1N1 after doing laboratory diagnostic tests. The researcher wants to use these medical records, the artifacts, to conduct the evaluation.

Since there is a large set of records, the researcher uses stratified sampling. It is known that 40% of recorded flu cases are H1N1 and so he randomly selects 400 records from the H1N1 group and 600 records from the other group. The researcher decided against using all medical records in this evaluation, so that sufficient unused records are available for later evaluations.

Choose the Dependent Variable

The dependent variables need to relate to the goal of the study and the algorithm. For example, the goal of including an algorithm in a decision support system can be to improve decision accuracy or to save time. Stating the goals and the hypotheses related to them will help identify the best dependent variables to measure. They should allow the researcher to make a conclusion about the hypotheses and thus about whether the goal was reached or not. For example, if the goal of the algorithm is to improve decision making, the hypotheses could be that the algorithm will be superior in terms of the number of correct decisions and the time needed to make the decisions compared to a system without the algorithm. The dependent variables measured in the study are naturally the number of correct decisions and the decision time.

Different types of sets with artifacts can be used. It is possible that in a set of artifacts, only one or a few represent the correct or best outcome. For example, when the algorithm completes a retrieval task, the researcher can use measures such as precision, true positive, true negative, sensitivity and specificity among others (see Part I – Chap. 2). However, if each artifact contains both the input and the required output of the algorithm, other measures are more appropriate. For example, definitive testing can provide the correct outcomes and that information is often part of the artifact, for example, with medical records containing mammograms and biopsy results. In this case, a measure such as accuracy of all decisions made using the algorithm is appropriate. Finally, artifacts can contain partial information about the answers or solutions, such as that found in a multitude of texts online. Then outcome measures should evaluate how correct and complete an answer is when provided by the algorithm.

Sometimes the set of artifacts available for evaluation is so large that it is impractical to use it in its entirety as a gold standard. This is the case when the correct solution depends on scoring each item in advance. When this is impossible, the scoring can be completed on an as-needed basis. For example, when evaluating whether an algorithm can retrieve images from a large set to match an example image, the entire set of available images cannot be evaluated in advance. The images need to be evaluated after applying the algorithm. To provide such scoring, precautions are necessary. The evaluators should be independent and different from the developers and should be blinded to the experimental conditions that produced the outcome.

In addition to the measures discussed above, there are also efficiency measures, such as runtime or memory usage, that are specifically used to evaluate algorithms. Most commonly, the processing time and memory usage are evaluated in relation to the size of the input using mathematical calculations, for example, the Big-O notation (see Part I – Chap. 2). These measures are related to how the algorithm runs and do not require a user study. Such evaluations are not the focus of the current recipe.

Applied Example

The company where the flu distinction algorithm was developed acquires the medical records for testing. This set of artifacts possesses the correct diagnosis for each case and so the following measures are chosen as the dependent variables: true positives, false positives, true negatives and false negatives. Sensitivity and specificity are also calculated. Such detailed assessment is important since assigning the wrong label has different consequences depending on the diseases being discussed. The metrics are also useful for comparisons with other approaches. In addition, the results will be published in the medical informatics field, where these are the expected measures. If the results were to be published in the computer science literature, the researcher would measure the same variables but would better present them as a confusion matrix.

Choose the Independent Variable

The independent variable defines how the new algorithm will be evaluated. The set of chosen conditions, including the new algorithm, forms the independent variable. When the algorithm is a novel approach, there are no other algorithms that can serve as a comparison point. One option for researchers would be to limit themselves to a description of system outcomes. However, it is much more interesting to compare the algorithm with existing conditions, without the algorithm, to demonstrate the usefulness of the algorithm. A user study comparing the algorithm with a well chosen baseline can accomplish this. Even when no comparable algorithms exist, there are several options to choose a baseline that do not require interaction between users and the algorithm.

A first possible baseline is a *lower bound* baseline. This is the minimum number of correct solutions that would be achieved without using the algorithm. A popular approach is the use of a majority case, where the most common outcome is assigned to all cases. The most common outcome is the one that has the highest chance of being correct. As an alternative to the majority case, a random outcome could be assigned. Algorithms should at least perform better than these baselines, since the baseline represents the outcome that can be achieved without any effort or algorithm.

In addition to a lower bound, the *human answer* could be used as a comparison point. In many cases, an algorithm is compared to how people performed without the algorithm. Experts or representative users can form the baseline and perform the tasks. The algorithm is compared against that outcome. For example, experts may provide 80% correct diagnoses and representative users such as non-expert clinicians may provide 68% correct diagnoses, while the algorithm provides 76% correct diagnoses. These are often the more interesting baselines against which to compare. They can also usually be established in advance and do not require the users to interact with the algorithm.

Note: in theory, an *upper bound* such as the perfect solution could also be included. The algorithm outcome could be compared against the 100% correct solution. However, this is indirectly already included when a gold standard is used: the outcome is calculated in relation to that perfect solution. Limiting the experiment to such a comparison would only provide one measure and not a comparison with other conditions without the algorithm.

Applied Example

The goal is to use this flu classification algorithm for diagnosis when no definitive testing is available, for example, based on a telephone interview. Therefore, a person's diagnosis based on the same limited information would be very valuable. This information is available as the initial diagnosis noted in the medical record, which was written down before definitive testing was conducted. The experiment will therefore compare two conditions of one independent variable: the algorithm's decision and the clinician's decision when the case was recorded.

There is a potential problem with this approach. The first diagnosis may not be available for all records. It can also be expected that an initial diagnosis was explicitly noted only when there was a clear indication for one type of flu or another. If only records with an initial diagnosis are included, it may show an accuracy rate not achieved when all records could have been used. As an alternative, the researcher could recruit an experienced nurse who would receive and review all records from which the laboratory tests are removed and assign one of two labels to each record: seasonal flu or H1N1 flu. As a result of this additional data collection, each medical record would have a human expert gold standard to compare against.

It is the researcher's task to balance the different options, taking potential bias into account as well as the practical aspects of the study. In this recipe, it is assumed there was no need to recruit a nurse and all medical records contained the necessary information.

Choose the Study Design

The simplest version of the study described in this recipe contains one independent variable with two conditions to compare the algorithm with another condition. A within-subjects design in this case is feasible, even when there are more than two conditions, because the data points for each condition do not come from people who are recruited and undergo a treatment. Instead, the data points come from artifacts, i.e., the data from people. These artifacts undergo the experimental conditions. As such, the people themselves are not involved anymore (at least not in person). This helps avoid many types of bias and simplifies the study design. In this aspect an informatics study is very different from typical studies in the behavioral sciences.

When using a within-subjects design, the same artifacts can be reused in all experimental conditions. The artifacts can be randomly sampled from all those available. Stratified sampling can be used when artifacts can be grouped in different classes, such as easy and difficult cases. Once the artifacts have been processed in the experimental conditions, the resulting scores for the dependent variable can be analyzed. When there are only two conditions and a within-subjects design is used, the paired samples t-test is appropriate. The data points in each condition are related to each other and form each other's baseline. When there are more than two conditions, a repeated measures ANOVA is the appropriate analysis. In this case, post hoc comparisons will be necessary when a significant effect has been found for the independent variable.

Because humans are not involved, several difficulties with user studies disappear and the study is much simpler to conduct. First, since multiple conditions can be tested on the same input artifacts, fewer artifacts are needed. In addition, there is no risk of tiring or boring subjects, there is no risk of a learning effect across conditions and there is no need to randomize the order of conditions. Naturally, other potential problems, such as experimenter bias, still need to be taken into account. For example, when experts evaluate the output of an algorithm or compile a gold standard as the reference point, care should be taken that no bias is introduced. It is preferable that the gold standard is compiled in advance; however, when this is impossible and the outcome is evaluated after application of the algorithms, care should be taken that the experts are blind to the experimental conditions.

Alternatively, the researchers may decide to use a between-subjects design, where each experimental condition uses different artifacts. In this case, more artifacts are needed so that each condition has sufficient data points. These can be randomly selected from the entire collection of artifacts, similar to the within-subjects design. This study design may be less powerful for detecting a small effect but it includes more types of artifacts and so the external validity is better. For this design, an independent samples *t*-test should be conducted when there are two conditions, or an ANOVA can be used for more than two conditions. Post hoc analysis is necessary when the ANOVA detects significant effects for variables with more than two conditions.

Applied Example

The researcher decides to use a within-subjects design, and a set of randomly selected medical records is used in both experimental conditions. Each record is processed by the algorithm, which is one condition of the independent variable. The original diagnosis included before definitive tests were conducted is also available and this forms the second condition of the independent variable. Since there is no risk of a carryover effect, the same records can be used in both conditions. Because there is a relationship between the data points in both conditions, the researcher will conduct a paired samples t-test.

Complete IRB Requirements

Although this recipe involves the evaluation of an algorithm without human involvement, there may be IRB requirements. Depending on the institution, funding origin and information included in the artifacts, the IRB requirements will be different. If IRB approval is necessary, the approval needs to be received before any evaluation activities commence. However, it is most likely that the artifacts will be exempt from review or qualify for expedited review.

It is essential to verify that the artifacts can be used for the study as intended. For some data, approval for its use for research purposes has already been collected. However, if this is not the case, approval may need to be acquired from subjects. The researcher should check how the artifacts were acquired and what the policies are for using them for research. The categories of data that can be used for research purposes were discussed in Part II – Chap. 5.

When using existing datasets, different rules can be expected for those with and without personal identification information. When using a public dataset that does not include such personal identification information, no IRB approval should be necessary. However, many institutions still require submission of the study. In other cases, some 'scrubbing' of data will be necessary to remove personal identifying information. With the increasing availability of user logs in different disciplines and awareness of the need to protect privacy, several data log scrubbing and privacy tools have been developed [2–4]. Regardless of these, most IRB processes will require the researcher to provide details on how the data will be treated and how privacy or confidentiality will be maintained.

Applied Example

The researcher completes the IRB process at the university that will supply the medical records. The application includes an explanation of how confidentiality of information will be maintained. This will be accomplished by not transferring personal identification information, such as contact information, with the medical records. Furthermore, procedures are established such that no data will be published that is not based on aggregate numbers to avoid the possibility that individuals could be recognized based on the combination of their submitted information.

Conduct the Study

Once all decisions have been made, the hard work is done. Researchers can execute the study, calculate the results and report the findings.

Note that it may save significant time with future work if all steps and decisions are written out in a detailed manner. This can form the basis for a detailed research protocol which, when finalized, research assistants can follow to conduct the study finalized. It could also then be repeated with other algorithms.

Applied Example

After completing all IRB requirements, the researcher randomly selects the medical records. Each record is submitted to the algorithm and, for each, the initial diagnosis is also recorded. For both conditions, the outcome is compared against the final diagnosis that is based on definitive tests. Based on this data, true positive, true negative, false positive and false negative are calculated for each condition, followed by sensitivity and specificity. For each dependent variable, the researcher conducts a paired samples t-test and compares the algorithm outcome with the initial diagnosis.

References

1. Cooper A (2008) A survey of query log privacy-enhancing techniques from a policy perspective. ACM Trans Web 2 (4):Article 19. doi:10.1145/1409220.1409222
2. Gonzales CK (2010) Eliciting user requirements using appreciative inquiry. Ph.D. dissertation, Claremont Graduate University
3. Huang L-C, Huei-ChungChu, Chung-YuehLien, Chia-HungHsiao, TsairKao (2009) Privacy preservation and information security protection for patients' portable electronic health records. Comput Biol Med 39(9):743–750
4. Uzuner O, Sibanda TC, Luo Y, Szolovits P (2008) A de-identifier for medical discharge summaries. Artif Intell Med 42(1):13–35

Recipe 2: Evaluating Standalone Algorithms Using Subjects

Recipe Summary

Figure A.2.1 shows the overview of the recipes discussed in this section and highlights where the current recipe fits. Similar to the previous recipe, this one discusses the evaluation of an algorithm by itself. It is assumed to be a novel algorithm for which no suitable comparison algorithm exists. However, this recipe demonstrates an evaluation with subjects taking part in the study. They will evaluate the output of the algorithm or complete tasks using the algorithm. A common study approach is to compare tasks that are solved by users with or without the help of the algorithm. User involvement is especially important for algorithms where user preferences, judgments or insights play an important role in the algorithm's ultimate usefulness.

Place in the Development Life Cycle and Example

As always, including testing and evaluation of algorithms early on will lead to a more robust information system. This is particularly crucial for algorithms that rely on user opinion, interaction or feedback. The performance of such algorithms is more difficult to predict since the intended users are typically very different from the developers and they will have different assumptions, expectations and preferences. Examples include data display and visualization algorithms; algorithms that interact with users, such as intelligent tutors, or rely on their feedback; and algorithms that offer suggestions or rankings.

The benefits of early testing also apply to this recipe: problems can be identified early on and their origin is easier to pinpoint. This makes it faster and cheaper to fix problems. The solutions themselves usually are better too since the algorithm has

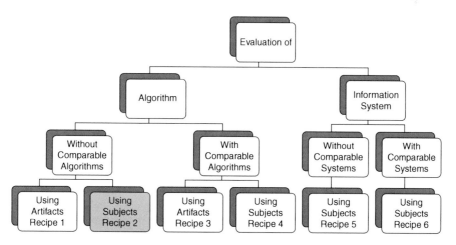

Fig. A.2.1 Standalone algorithm evaluation using subjects

not yet been integrated with other components. An additional advantage of working with people early on is that more diverse responses can be expected. This makes it possible to adjust the system to a greater diversity of views and preferences which will benefit the final product.

For the current recipe, it is assumed that there are tasks that need to be completed that require the algorithm to interact with the user. Even so, the evaluation can focus on algorithms that independently solve problems or algorithms that assist users in their tasks. Most algorithms in this category will replace an entire process or part of the process that historically was completed by people.

Applied Example

In this chapter, the following fictitious example is used to illustrate individual steps.

Researchers who tackle a new problem are confronted with the need to read hundreds of papers and other relevant materials containing the necessary background information. This is especially the case in biomedicine where the number of publications increases enormously – exponentially for some topics [1, 2]. Reading and digesting the information is a lifelong process. Many algorithms are being developed in informatics to support and facilitate such activities. One example is the development of an algorithm that combines information from the literature with experiment data. More specifically, when a researcher submits the results of an experiment, the algorithm is intended to automatically find supporting and contradictory evidence in the literature. The researcher who developed this has used its results for her own research but now wants to evaluate whether it also would be useful for others.

Choose the Dataset

The data in this evaluation will be based on input to the algorithm which is processed. Either the resulting output or the process to get the output is the subject of the evaluation by users. Similar to other evaluations, the input used for the algorithm cannot have been used during the development phases. Such reuse would result in an overestimate of the capability of the algorithm since the algorithm will have been tuned and optimized to process it.

It is ideal if a large set of inputs, usually artifacts, is available from which a random selection can be made for the study. If all are in the same style, difficulty level or generally share the same characteristics, a simple random selection suffices. If there are classes in the input data, such as simple and complex items, then a stratified sampling is more appropriate.

The size of the dataset needed and the number of users needed depend on the design of the study. A rule of thumb is to have 30 or more data points in each experimental condition. Since people are involved in this recipe's evaluation, the input cannot be used in multiple conditions if that would lead to second look bias. For example, if the input is a task that users complete on their own and also with support of an algorithm, the task should be different in each condition to prevent learning or other carryover effects from one condition to the next. The number of such input items will further depend on the number of users involved. Each user can complete multiple tasks if they are short, which requires more different artifacts. If each participant works on one task, fewer artifacts will be needed, but more participants will need to be recruited to get to the optimal number of data points for the study.

Applied Example

Since the new algorithm can support many activities, there are different options on how to conduct its evaluations. The researcher decides to first focus on "literature review at the start of new research" and adjusts the scope of the study to this process. This task was chosen because it represents a single task that is always part of a more comprehensive literature review. The dataset needed to evaluate this will consist of queries that would be submitted to search engines and digital libraries. The result of processing these queries will be the base for the evaluation. Since it is difficult to artificially create such queries, the researcher works with a group of first-year graduate students in the biology department. She chooses them since they conduct experiments as part of their courses and need to learn all about these topics from the literature. By choosing to work with graduate students, the researcher has limited the scope of her study to a group of beginning researchers.

Note that the scope of the study is limited to a particular group and particular problem. This will allow for clear conclusions since it will be easier to avoid confounding among variables. However, as a consequence, the conclusions will be limited to that user group and that problem.

Choose the Dependent Variable

The dependent variable should be chosen to reflect the goal of the study. Since the evaluation in this recipe is conducted with subjects and not artifacts, there are different options for conducting it. As always, it is helpful to restate the goal of the study and the associated hypotheses. The dependent variables need to be chosen so they allow the researcher to accept or reject the hypotheses.

In general, two types of evaluations can be conducted and combined when people are involved: an objective and a subjective evaluation of the algorithm. The objective evaluation relies on measures that allow assessment of the algorithm outcome. The correct solution must be available, either based on definitive tests or another type of gold standard. Measures such as accuracy, true positives, time delay and others are then calculated in each experimental condition (see Part I – Chap. 2).

A second set of outcome measures is also possible: subjective measures. Study subjects can be queried about their opinion and experience completing the tasks with and without the algorithm. For example, they can be queried on the difficulty of completing the task, how confident they are about their answer and the usability. When subjects participate in multiple experimental conditions, they can be asked to compare the different experiences.

Standard evaluations that look at runtime or resources needed by the algorithms are not applicable to this experiment. However, time to completion can be a fitting measure when it focuses on the time needed by subjects to complete the tasks.

Applied Example

Since this algorithm is intended to support people, the researcher decides to include both objective and subjective measurements. Her goal is to compare the completeness of a literature review, how much time can be saved by using the algorithm and how well people can work with the algorithm.

To measure the completeness of the literature review, the researcher will count the number of PubMed abstracts that are found relevant to the course experiment. To decide on the relevance of the lists of abstracts, she will work with the faculty member who assigned the course project and is up to date on the related literature. However, because this course faculty member knows the individual students, the researcher will need to be careful to avoid bias when the results are evaluated (see Conduct the Study). The students will measure the time taken by keeping a log of their time. This will be a coarse measure of time taken. If a more fine-grained measure was necessary, the researcher could opt to include software-based tracking. However, since a difference of a few seconds or minutes does not matter with a literature review, the log will suffice. The subjective measures consist of a short Likert scale to measure how easy subjects felt it was to complete the tasks and how confident they are that they have a complete review of the literature.

Choose the Independent Variable

The independent variable defines the different conditions of the study. In most informatics studies, an experiment will contain one or two independent variables. One independent variable focuses on comparing the new algorithm with another condition. This comparison should relate the study back to its original goals. For example, if the goal of the algorithm is to help people make better decisions, a comparison should be made of decisions with and without the algorithm. When there is only one such comparison condition, it is often referred to as a baseline. In many studies, the independent variable will contain more than two conditions, for example, a condition without an algorithm, a condition with the basic algorithm and a condition with a more advanced algorithm.

While the previous recipe (where only artifacts were used) discussed comparing performance with an upper and lower bound, this recipe focuses on usefulness of the algorithm to users. A natural baseline is therefore a condition where users do not have algorithm support which is compared to users with algorithm support. This comparison can be executed with or without a gold standard to measure against. If a gold standard is available, it will allow measures such as accuracy and will also show how closely the outcome of each experimental condition, with and without algorithm support, approaches the perfect solution.

Applied Example

The researcher decides to compare the new algorithm with a baseline condition without the algorithm. In her case, this means comparing how completely and efficiently a literature review can be conducted with (Condition 1) and without (Condition 2) the algorithm. Each student in the class receives the same research problem and experiment to conduct. After agreeing to participate in the study, half of the students are randomly selected to work with the new algorithm while the other half work without an algorithm.

Naturally, students working with the algorithm will receive a tutorial on how to use it. To avoid bias, the researcher decides that both groups of students will receive a tutorial: one group on how to work with the algorithm and the other group (baseline) on how to work with the normal online resources that this university offers. Both tutorials will be equal in length and use the same approach and examples.

Choose the Study Design

The study will contain at least one independent variable where the algorithm is compared to a baseline condition without the algorithm. In this case, the independent variable has two conditions. However, more conditions can also be included. For example, there may be multiple versions of the algorithm. Naturally, additional independent variables can also be included, for example, the different types of users may be of scientific or business interest. The data points in each condition will now depend on the number of subjects and the number of artifacts or tasks they can complete. For each experimental condition, the researcher will need sufficient data points to show statistical differences when they exist.

When people are involved, there are many types of bias that can influence the results. While the design of this study is straightforward, the optimal choices are different when people, not artifacts, are directly involved as subjects. The researcher should carefully consider which biases may be at play and can be controlled when choosing between a within- or between-subjects design. For example, carryover effects need to be considered with within-subjects designs; history effects need to be considered with between-subjects designs. In addition, since this recipe focuses on working with people, other common sources of unwanted variances may be: domain knowledge, experience, age and gender, among others.

If the researcher chooses a within-subjects design for an independent variable, the subjects will participate in all conditions of that independent variable. In this case, the order of the conditions should be randomized for each subject to avoid carryover or other ordering effects. For example, when there are two conditions, half of the subjects should receive one order and the other half of the subjects should receive another order. The most appropriate analysis to be conducted is a paired samples t-test for experiments with only one independent variable with two conditions. With more conditions or more variables, ANOVA is the appropriate analysis. Repeated measures ANOVA should be used for the within-subjects variable. When there are more than two conditions, post hoc analysis will be needed for variables that should have a significant effect.

The researcher can also choose to conduct the study as a between-subjects experiment. In this case, a different group of subjects will participate in the different conditions of the experiment. Random assignment should be used to assign a subject to a condition. The experimental conditions should be conducted as close together in time as possible to avoid history effects. When there are only two conditions, an independent samples t-test is the most appropriate analysis. When there are more conditions or more than one variable, an ANOVA should be conducted, followed by post hoc comparisons if a significant effect is found. This design may be less powerful than a within-subjects design since more variance can be expected in the groups. The subjects are different in each experimental condition and do not serve as their own baseline. However, in many cases, this design is more practical to carry out and avoids learning effects or other types of carryover effects.

Applied Example

Since each group of students participates in one experimental condition, a between-subjects design is followed. There are almost 100 students in this course who all agreed to participate. Each student is randomly assigned to one of the two conditions of the independent variable (algorithm or not). Once the experiment is completed, the researcher has data for several dependent variables, such as the number of abstracts found, the time taken and the subjective evaluations. For each of these dependent variables, the researcher will conduct an independent samples t-test.

Complete IRB Requirements

The researcher should check with her institution on the IRB requirements. It is best to start this process early since it may take several weeks before an approval is received. It is also common for the IRB to require clarifications or changes in the study setup. All previous steps will need to be explained in the IRB documents. The study cannot commence until approval has been received.

Common requirements for IRB approval are an explanation of the goal of the study, the study design, how subjects will be recruited and how the data will be collected, stored and analyzed. The researcher also needs to consider and explain how confidentiality will be provided. In many cases, consideration must be given to the consequences of participating and ensuring there are no additional consequences. For example, when conducted in a work environment, performance in the study should be confidential and should not influence work performance reviews. Since few IRB members will have computational experience, care should be taken to include a layman's explanation of the algorithm.

The algorithm is really the subject of the study; it is what is being evaluated. However, IRB requirements will still need to be completed since there are people involved. It is helpful to explain this difference between evaluations in informatics and in behavioral sciences in the introduction of the IRB application since the evaluation of informatics studies is not yet a mainstream activity in most universities. Using the term 'participants' rather than 'subjects', is one way to emphasize that the algorithms are the focus of the study, not the people.

Applied Example

The researcher checks her institution's policy and submits an application that explains the study details, the recruitment procedures and how data will be collected and analyzed. The application also includes a letter from the course faculty member stating that he agrees that students will be recruited in his course.

As often happens, the IRB members have concerns about the effects of the study on the university students who will be participating. They require that the researcher explain how students will be recruited, how they can opt out of the study, how she will ensure there are no consequences of participating or not and how it can be ensured that everyone in the course has a similar chance of getting a good grade. To address the issue of grades, it is decided, in discussion with the course faculty member, to add a debriefing at the end of the study and provide all students, regardless of experimental condition, with a tutorial on how to use the university resources and the new algorithm and also give them sufficient time to improve their literature review. This ensures that no students receive an unfair advantage. These changes are included in the design and the revision submitted to the IRB, which then later approves the study.

Conduct the Study

Once all decisions have been made and IRB approval received, the study is executed. While interacting with the IRB, practical aspects of the study can be completed, such as printing worksheets and finding and reserving rooms. Once the study has been completed, the data can be evaluated and analyzed.

Often, recruiting a sufficiently large group of users to participate takes a long time. Therefore many studies are conducted with students, who form a convenient subject pool. Care should be taken, however, that these subjects are representative of the intended users.

Applied Example

Students are recruited by the researcher, who explains the study, and the course faculty member, who explains how the fairness of their grade is ensured. Then, the researcher hands out a sign-up sheet. Students who participate are randomly assigned to a condition and then invited to the tutorial session for their condition, followed by a work session. Students are not told whether they receive the baseline or experimental tutorial. They receive free movie tickets when they complete the study. They are required to submit their findings to the researcher at the end of the work session. This avoids communication between students about the experiment. In their course, all students, whether they participated in the study or not, receive a tutorial on how to do a literature search and are invited to use the different available resources.

The results have only a study participant number associated with them. Each of these numbers has been associated in advance with the experimental conditions (random assignment). All PubMed abstracts that make up the results are combined and duplicates are removed. The course faculty member receives this list and evaluates it as appropriate or not. Based on this list, the individual results of study participants are then calculated and each receives a score based on the number of relevant abstracts found. In addition, the subjective evaluations are compiled. Statistical testing is done for each dependent variable.

References

1. Leroy G, Fiszman M, Rindflesch TC (2008) The impact of directionality in predications on text mining. Hawaii International Conference on System Sciences, 7–10 Jan 2008
2. Perutz MF (1999) Will biomedicine outgrow support? Nature 399:299–301

Recipe 3: Comparing Algorithms Using Artifacts

Recipe Summary

Figure A.3.1 shows how this recipe discusses the evaluation of an algorithm in comparison to another algorithm or other versions of the algorithm. The algorithm processes artifacts, i.e., records, images or any other type of man-made object, and can be evaluated without interaction with its future users. The recipe is similar to the first recipe, since the set of artifacts contains the correct answer or can be used to calculate the correct answer; however, here the goal of the study is to compare the performance of the new algorithm to the performance of another. It is essential to choose a valid baseline, and researchers should be careful not to work with demo versions of algorithms or default values when those are not appropriate. Study designs in this category are often simpler than those in the behavioral sciences because there is no direct interaction with people which means there is less danger of bias that can influence the results.

Place in the Development Life Cycle

This evaluation is necessary when a new algorithm has been developed that focuses on a problem or tasks for which there already are computational solutions. The algorithm that needs to be evaluated can be compared against another algorithm or another version of the algorithm. A main advantage of evaluating an algorithm early on is that any problems can be caught and fixed before it is integrated in the information system. This makes it easier to pinpoint the problems and correct them. At this point in the development cycle, it also is cheaper to make the necessary changes.

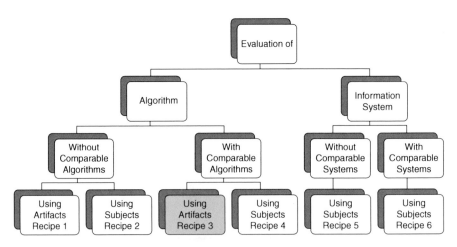

Fig. A.3.1 Algorithm comparison using artifacts

Although early testing may seem to slow down the development process, it will lead to better and more robust algorithms.

When conducting an evaluation by using an existing set of artifacts, as in this recipe, it is somewhat easier to conduct an objective evaluation compared to working with people directly. Moreover, when working with an individual algorithm instead of a complete information system, it is usually easier to create such a set of artifacts. Unfortunately, comparing a new algorithm with other existing algorithms also may pose problems. One such problem is that the comparison algorithms need to be carefully chosen so that conclusions drawn from the study are meaningful. A second potential problem is that the existing comparison algorithms may already be included in another, complete information system making a direct comparison difficult.

The type of evaluation in this recipe is typical in medicine where new approaches are often only accepted when it has been shown they provide an advantage over established approaches. For this recipe, it is assumed that a set of artifacts that contains the input required by the algorithm exists or can be created, as well as the perfect, approved or best possible solution. The artifacts can be of many different types, ranging from wet lab experiment output that needs to be clustered to images or numeric data or even online communities that need to be mined. Similar to evaluating a new algorithm on its own (Recipe 1), multiple evaluations can be done when the dataset is sufficiently large. For example, Leroy et al. [1] evaluated different versions of a word sense disambiguation algorithm for medical text by comparing each version against an expert created gold standard. The different versions of the algorithms used increasingly more information. The artifacts, words in sentences, were reused in the different conditions.

Applied Example

In this chapter, the following fictitious example will be used to illustrate each step.

> A researcher in computational linguistics has been working on a parser to automatically extract all gene and protein names from text. The parser contains several components, including a tokenizer which identifies individual words; a part-of-speech tagger which assigns the part of speech to each word, such as noun, adjective, verb; and an entity extraction algorithm that identifies which nouns are genes or proteins. The entity extraction algorithm is the focus of the evaluation. The new algorithm is rule-based and is an improved version of an earlier approach to algorithmically extract genes and proteins from text. This first version was tested using 150 biomedical abstracts and achieved high precision (94%) but low recall (43%). The researcher has been working on improvements to increase the recall. He decided to make the rules less strict so that more words are recognized as representing a gene or protein. Ideally, this happens without decreasing precision but a study will need to be done to make sure.

Choose the Dataset

Similar to evaluating an algorithm by itself, a set of artifacts needs to be made available or created for the evaluation of multiple algorithms. Naturally, the artifacts selected for the evaluation need to be different from those used during development of the algorithms. Especially when comparing with other algorithms, reusing data would provide an unfair advantage to the algorithms that were developed using that particular data.

The set of artifacts selected should be large enough to allow a statistical comparison between the results of the different conditions. Use the rule of thumb which means that there should be 30 or more data points in each experimental condition. Keep in mind that the number 30 is only a guideline. With strong experimental effects a smaller number may suffice, but with a small experimental effect more may be needed to detect a statistically significant difference.

To evaluate algorithms without human involvement, there are often large sets of artifacts available that can be used in the study without practically hampering its execution. This is not so when people have to be recruited to participate. An advantage of including more artifacts is that the study will have more power. In addition, there will probably be better external validity since a larger variety of input is most likely a better representation of what can be expected beyond the scope of a single study. Ideally, the set of artifacts is big enough so that a large, random selection can be made of those artifacts to be included in the study.

Sometimes, the available set of artifacts can be so large that it is unnecessary or not possible to include all data. If that is the case, a subset of items to be used in the evaluation can be randomly selected. If the dataset contains classes of artifacts, a stratified sample can be taken. Keep in mind that when comparing between different versions of an algorithm or between different algorithms, the intent is to show a statistical difference. With more data points, the study has more power and will be more likely to detect differences if they exist.

For evaluations of algorithms without human involvement, a different type of evolution is possible when a large dataset is available: n-fold cross-validation (see Part I – Chap. 2). It is appropriate to evaluate machine learning algorithms and often included with the software [2]. With this evaluation, the dataset is divided into n subsets of which $n-1$ are used for training a model and one set is used for testing. This process is repeated n times so that each subset serves once as the test set. The outcome for the tests is averaged. This evaluation is common for standalone machine learning approaches, but it is less suitable when comparing two approaches with each other using statistical analysis. This is because n-fold cross-validation returns only one data point for each algorithm (or condition): the average performance, usually accuracy, over the n-folds. Thus, statistical testing cannot be performed.

Applied Example

From the previous evaluation, the researcher possesses a large dataset with 150 biomedical abstracts of journal articles discussing genes and proteins. However, after the first evaluation the researcher used this dataset to improve the rules that make up the algorithm. Therefore, using these abstracts for a formal comparison between the old and new algorithm is inappropriate and a new dataset containing other biomedical abstracts is needed. In each abstract, all genes and proteins need to be identified. This set of abstracts will become the new gold standard to be used in the study. To construct this gold standard, a biomedical expert is recruited who reads a set of 100 biomedical abstracts in his domain of expertise. This expert tags all genes and proteins in each abstract. Only one expert is engaged for creating this gold standard since it is expected that there would be little or no variation in tagging between two experts. The standard can therefore be expected to be general and not limited to the single expert's opinion.

Choose the Dependent Variable

The dependent variable should be related to the goal of the study and allow a researcher to evaluate the algorithms based on those variables. If the new algorithm provides an improvement, this will show in differences in values for those variables. The artifacts can usually be reused in the different experimental conditions since this recipe focuses on a comparison of algorithms without direct user interaction.

The choice of dependent variables depends on the available artifacts. Similar to standalone algorithm evaluations, when the dataset is made up of artifacts of which some are the answer to a task or question, the evaluations should focus on verifying that algorithms discover that artifact. Measures such as precision, true positives or true negatives can be used. If each artifact in the dataset contains the required outcome or it can be calculated, for example, with results from definitive tests, then the result of applying the algorithm on a subset of artifacts can be compared with the included correct answers. In this case, measures such as accuracy can be calculated. Finally, when artifacts provide partial solutions or answers, the dependent variable can be focused on completeness of answers with a measure such as recall.

Sometimes it is impractical to define the correct answer in advance because of the size of the dataset. For example, when evaluating a search engine for a collection of ten million articles, it is not practical to score every possible article for different possible user queries. In this case, the results will need to be evaluated after executing the algorithm. If the evaluation relies on a human answer, a few additional precautions are necessary. The first is that the evaluators should be different from the developers and should be representative, as much as possible, of the final users. A second precaution is that the evaluators should be blind to the experimental conditions. This means that they should not be aware which algorithm was the origin of the output. The best approach to accomplish this is to combine the output from all algorithms that are being evaluated into one set. Then the order of the output items should be randomized. The experimenter should explain this process to the evaluators to avoid bias towards one algorithm or another. With a random order and without knowledge of the condition the outcome belongs to, the evaluation will be more objective.

Naturally, the evaluation of algorithms can also focus on their efficiency and look at processing time, memory or power usage. Efficiency evaluations of algorithms can include calculations of the runtime and memory usage for different input sizes, such has the Big-O notation (see Part I – Chap. 2). In addition, runtimes can also be captured on a different scale, for example, to verify if waiting or loading times are acceptable and allow for good job performance by the future users. For example, calculations and visualization of 3D or live video, such as video of living organs, will depend on memory and processing power, but in telemedicine, other factors such as the type of network connection and type of network will also affect the quality of the algorithms.

Applied Example

To evaluate whether the new algorithm is better than its older version in extracting gene and protein names from text, the researcher decides to calculate precision and recall of gene and protein names. This is done by comparing the genes and proteins identified by the algorithm with those identified by the expert. A set of biomedical abstracts not yet used during development was randomly selected. Care was taken that these abstracts were in the expert's domain of expertise. Then, all genes and proteins were identified in advance by the expert. Based on this gold standard, the outcome measures will be calculated. Precision measures the percentage of terms identified by the algorithm that are genes and proteins, while recall is the percentage of all required genes and proteins that were identified by the algorithm.

Choose the Independent Variable

When two or more algorithms are being compared, there will be minimally one independent variable in the experiment reflecting these algorithms. Each algorithm will make up one condition of that independent variable. When an established algorithm is compared with a new algorithm, the established algorithm is usually referred to as the baseline for comparison. The new algorithm will be compared against this baseline.

When multiple versions of the same algorithm are being evaluated, each algorithm is seen as one condition for the independent variable. It is logical to choose the simplest version as the baseline. This is particularly true when there is also a rationale for the different versions of the algorithms, for example, they could use increasingly more data or increasingly more sophisticated functions. Then, such a choice of baseline is logical.

Naturally, when there are other variables of interest, the study can contain additional independent variables. For example, when testing generic text processing algorithms that are intended to work for all Germanic languages, an additional independent variable could be chosen for the different languages. For example, Afrikaans, English, German and Swedish could each form one condition of that second independent variable.

Applied Example

The researcher is only interested in English language abstracts and so he includes only one independent variable in his study which focuses on the algorithm that is being applied. This independent variable has two conditions: the old algorithm which serves as the baseline and the new, improved algorithm.

Choose the Study Design

In this recipe, algorithms are being compared using artifacts without direct interaction with users. Similar to evaluating a standalone algorithm, comparing different algorithms can be done with a simple study design. Usually, a within-subjects approach can be used where the same artifacts are used in the different experimental conditions. Since the artifacts, not people, are tested under the conditions, there is less potential for bias to distort the results. This feature of studies in informatics is different from studies in most other fields where people are studied, not algorithms or information systems.

For studies applying a within-subjects design, the same artifacts are used in all conditions. When there is only one independent variable with two conditions, a paired samples t-test is the most appropriate analysis. This t-test is appropriate because there is a relation between the data points in the two conditions: the artifacts are the same in both conditions. When there are more than two conditions or more than one independent variable, a repeated measures ANOVA is the most appropriate analysis. In this case, post hoc comparisons will be needed for the variable with a significant effect to pinpoint which conditions are significantly different from each other.

With large datasets, researchers may prefer to use different artifacts in the different experimental conditions and so apply a between-subjects design. They can randomly sample a number of artifacts from the dataset for each experimental condition. With one variable and two conditions, an independent samples t-test is the most appropriate analysis. With more than two conditions or more than one independent variable, an ANOVA should be conducted. Significant effects need to be followed up with post hoc analysis.

Similar to other recipes, there can be multiple independent variables that each follow different design principles. One variable can be tested with a within-subjects design while another uses a between-subjects design. Statistical software allows researcher to specify the approach for the variables. For example, when different text processing algorithms are tested, a second independent variable could be the language of the text. Since German text may differ from French text for many features, a between-subjects design could be used for language and a within-subjects design for the different algorithms.

Applied Example

The researcher first collects new abstracts for his evaluation. For each abstract, the genes and proteins are identified in advance by the expert. Since he is comparing two algorithms, he uses a within-subjects design and will conduct a paired samples t-test.

Complete IRB Requirements

Similar to all evaluations of algorithms that rely on data created by humans, the researcher should check the policy of the institution where the research takes place. When submitting IRB information, the characteristics of the dataset will play a role.

If it is public and does not contain personal identification information, the IRB approval process may be unnecessary. If there is personal identification information, the researchers can try to remove this in advance. In this case, some IRB review may be necessary. If personal identification information is part of the dataset, IRB review will be required but will most likely be expedited.

When IRB review is required, the goal and procedures of the study need to be explained. In addition, the researchers need to explain where and how the dataset will be collected and how personal identification information is treated, protected and published.

Applied Example

The researcher works with biomedical abstracts from which entities, genes and proteins, are extracted. One biomedical expert tags all abstracts. This study does not require IRB approval since no human subjects are involved and the artifacts, in this case the abstracts, are in the public domain and do not contain personal identification information.

Conduct the Study

A significant amount of work has been completed once all decisions have been made. If an IRB review was necessary, approval needs to be received before the study can commence. Then, researchers can execute the study and report the results. This means that algorithms need to be prepared to process the artifacts. Depending on the evaluation chosen, the outcomes may be automatically evaluated or manually compared with a gold standard or required outcome.

Once the algorithms have been applied and the outcome evaluated, statistical tests are conducted. The correct tests need to be selected based on the study design chosen. If more than two conditions have been tested and a significant main effect is found, post hoc comparisons need to be conducted to pinpoint the conditions that significantly differ.

Applied Example

The researcher randomly selected the biomedical abstracts to be used in the evaluation. These abstracts were sent to the biomedical expert who tagged each abstract and indicated which phrases in the text are genes or proteins. Meanwhile, the researcher applies both versions of the algorithm to the abstracts. For each abstract, the genes and proteins extracted by the algorithm are compared with those identified by the biomedical expert. For each abstract, precision and recall is calculated. This dataset is then used as the basis for a paired samples t-test. The results showed that the improvements made to the algorithms paid off, and the recall was significantly higher for the new algorithm, while precision remained the same and no statistical difference was found.

References

1. Leroy G, Rindflesh TC (2005) Effects of Information and machine learning algorithms on word sense disambiguation with small datasets. Int J Med Inform 74(7–8):573–585
2. Witten IH, Frank E (2000) Data mining: practical machine learning tools and techniques with Java. The Morgan Kaufmann series in data management systems. Morgan Kaufmann, San Francisco

Recipe 4: Comparing Algorithms Using Subjects

Recipe Summary

As shown in Fig. A.4.1, this recipe discusses the evaluation of different algorithms based on user interaction. Similar to the previous chapter, two or more algorithms are compared with each other. However, in this recipe the evaluation requires interaction with users, who will evaluate and compare the output of the algorithms. A user evaluation is essential for algorithms that form a critical component of an information system and depend on user opinions. Both within- and between-subjects designs are common in this scenario. Naturally, since people are directly involved in the study, additional precautions will need to be taken to avoid bias so that the study has good internal validity. The tasks, environment and type of users participating in the study will affect the external validity.

Place in the Development Life Cycle

The early testing and evaluation of algorithms leads to more robust information systems. Evaluation with representative users is crucial for algorithms that depend on users' subjective expectations, opinions and preferences. With such algorithms, it can be expected that the developers' mental models will be different from the intended users, and formally evaluating the algorithms will help correct this and increase their usefulness.

There are many benefits to testing algorithms. First, the ability to find and solve problems earlier reduces the cost and difficulty of correcting problems. With algorithms that depend on users for input and on their evaluation of its output, the user study can catch misinterpretations, incorrect defaults or assumptions early in the development process. In addition, when algorithms have not yet been integrated into

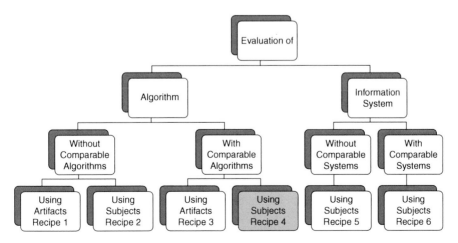

Fig. A.4.1 Algorithm comparison using subjects

the information system, any changes in the algorithm will have fewer implications for other components. Furthermore, when comparing multiple algorithms, the evaluation can show whether differences in algorithms have an impact. It is essential to conduct these studies when a new approach needs to be superior to older approaches.

For this recipe, it is assumed that there are datasets or tasks that can be entirely completed by algorithms or where the algorithms assist users in completing them. This recipe assumes the existence of another algorithm that will serve as a baseline or comparison point. The algorithms being evaluated are also assumed to be essential components of an information system that requires user interaction.

Applied Example

In this chapter, the following fictitious example will be used to illustrate each step.

> A software developer is building a new data mining toolkit to help cancer researchers discover interactions between genes and proteins. The algorithms, such as neural networks and support vector machines, predict up and down regulation of genes. The intended users are biomedical researchers. The algorithms are well known, and the focus of the toolkit is on visualization of the genes and proteins, the predictions of up and down regulation and the origin of the predictions. The origin of a prediction is important because each algorithm has its own estimated prediction accuracy. In addition, predictions are often based on combining the different algorithms using a voting scheme. A previous version of the software used a user interface that showed a network of genes and required that researchers click any link to see additional information. The interface was considered difficult to use. The new interface uses newer visualization algorithms, such as a spring algorithm to provide better positioning, and gives a better, consistent layout which visualizes the data using colors, line thickness and other symbols so that very limited additional clicking is required to get all information. The goal is to run an experiment to confirm that the new interface is better.

Choose the Dataset

The data in this evaluation will be based on the input submitted to and processed by the algorithms. Users will process these artifacts with the support of the algorithms or they will evaluate the algorithms' output. As such, the process itself or the outcome is the subject of the users' evaluation. Since users are involved, it is essential that the input is realistic and representative of future use. It is even better if it is also interesting to the study participants, since that will make it easier to recruit and retain the participants. The input used in the study should be different from that used during earlier development and testing of any of the algorithms. Reusing it would overestimate the capabilities and efficiency of the algorithms that have been tuned for it.

When there is large dataset with possible input that is suitable for the study, random selection can be used. In many cases, there will be classes in the dataset, for example, easy and difficult problems, and then stratified random sampling can be used so that a representative number of cases are included from each such group.

The number of data points should be large enough to allow for a statistical comparison. The researcher needs to choose to work with many different inputs, many different users or both. The more diverse the input and users, the more general the conclusions can be. If only one task or data input is used per condition with 30 different users, the conclusions will be limited. Similarly, if one user participates and works with 30 tasks, the conclusions will similarly be limited. It is best to have multiple tasks or inputs and a variety of users. The exact number will depend on the design chosen for the study. Ideally, 30 or more data points will be available in each experimental condition. More data is needed to detect significant differences when the effect size is small. Fewer than 30 data points may suffice for larger effect sizes.

When subjects take part in multiple conditions, different tasks or input may be needed in each condition to avoid carryover effects between experimental conditions. When subjects only take part in one experimental condition, the tasks or input items can be reused in each condition. In this case, the artifacts will be reused, but the users will be different. In addition, since users will be involved in this study, the difficulty level of the tasks or data, duration of the study and the type of user participating will need to be taken into account.

Applied Example

The developer works with two biomedical researchers who provide datasets of several experiments used to teach graduate students. Such experiments contain data that is easily understood by researchers in the field and so will not require significant learning by study participants. Each such dataset serves as one input to the algorithm. The developer plans to use a study design where each participant will evaluate both algorithms; therefore, he needs several experiments of comparable size and complexity to be divided over the two conditions. The resulting input in each condition used to test the visualization algorithms will be similar but from different experiments. At a minimum, two problems are needed per participant: one for each experimental condition. Then, each problem could be shown in an experimental condition to 30 or more study participants. However, because it is difficult to recruit enough users to participate, the developer plans on showing each user two problems per condition so that more data can be collected per participant.

Choose the Dependent Variable

The choice of dependent variable should reflect the goal of the algorithm and the study. The study should allow the researcher to conclude whether the algorithm accomplished its goal. With algorithms that require user interaction or input, the goal is usually broader than simple efficiency. As a result, several dependent variables will be relevant and will need to be considered for inclusion in the study.

A comparison of algorithms that relies on user interaction can use and combine objective and subjective measures. The objective measures will rely on metrics to evaluate the algorithm's outcomes (see Part I – Chap. 2), such as a count of tasks completed, answers to questions or solutions to problems. For this type of evaluation, the correct solution, a gold standard, needs to be available for all the tasks that are used in the study.

In addition to objective measures, subjective evaluations can be included. Study participants can be asked about their opinion on the use and usefulness of each algorithm after using it. Such a subjective evaluation can use multiple items to get a broad idea of the strengths and weaknesses of each algorithm. Depending on the user tasks, more detailed questions can be posed that focus on subtasks. When users interact with all algorithms that are being evaluated, they can be asked about their preference. Naturally, this should be asked after participants have had a chance to work with each algorithm.

Standard evaluations that look at runtime or resources needed by the algorithms are not very applicable to this type of study. Time to completion or the number of tasks completed in a limited time period are suitable alternatives. They are measures of time that will matter to intended users.

Applied Example

The developer has several choices for the dependent variable. The algorithms are intended to support researchers in their review of biomedical data. To this end, it is important that the data visualization provides an easy to understand overview of all the data with enough flexibility to show more or less detail, that it does not require a long learning period before the interface can be used and that researchers can easily distinguish between facts from experiments and predictions by machine learning algorithms.

The developer designs several multiple choice questions that focus on the users' understanding of the overall data, the details, and the difference between fact and prediction. The questions are presented on the same computer on which the visualization is tested and answers are recorded automatically. In addition, the time to completion is measured to get an idea of how long it takes to complete a task. This can be done by keeping track of the system time when the study was started and when the questions are answered. A more fine-grained time measurement is unnecessary since understanding and interpreting experiment data is not a task that biomedical researchers need to perform against the clock. However, with an easier-to-use interface, some time gain is expected. In each condition, a short survey will be presented using a 5-point Likert scale to ask participants their opinion of the algorithm. Example questions are: (1) it was easy to see all the genes and proteins measured, (2) it was easy to distinguish between the data (facts) and predictions, (3) it was clear how accurate the predictions were estimated to be … Finally, at the end of the study the participants also are asked if they prefer one of the algorithm to do a variety of tasks.

Choose the Independent Variable

Studies in informatics contain at least one independent variable to compare the different algorithms or information systems. When multiple algorithms are compared, they will usually form the different conditions of one independent variable; for example, with increasingly sophisticated algorithms each version can form one condition of the independent variable. It is important to choose reasonable algorithms for comparison and use them as intended. Care should be taken that the algorithms are not limited to demonstration versions which may not include all functionality or that they are not using unsuitable default values.

Naturally, there can be multiple independent variables. For example, both the approach and the amount of information used could each form an independent variable. The choice of independent variables should reflect the goal of the study so that, after conducting the study, researchers can draw conclusions about the different algorithms and how well they achieved their goal.

This recipe is different from a standalone evaluation of algorithms because each condition of the study will make use of an algorithm. If there is a logical relation between algorithms, then a baseline can be defined. For example, when a new, improved algorithm is compared against an older version, the latter can be considered a baseline. With increasingly sophisticated algorithms, the simplest one can be seen as the baseline. Regardless of this baseline, the evaluation remains the same when two or more algorithms are compared with each other.

Applied Example

The independent variable is very easy for the developer to define. It will be the algorithmic approach and it has two conditions: the old and the new algorithm. The new algorithm is expected to be superior to the old one for all types of input.

Choose the Study Design

This recipe focuses on the evaluation of algorithms that interact or depend on users. Because people are directly involved in the study, potential sources of bias and confounding variables need to be taken into account such as, learning effects and experimenter effects, among others. Depending on how well these can be controlled, the researcher can choose to apply a within-subjects or between-subjects design. For each variable, the choice between the two needs to be made. It is possible to mix the within- and between-subjects variables in one study.

In addition to taking bias into account, there need to be sufficient data points to make a statistical comparison possible. The number of data points and the statistical analysis will depend on the design that is chosen. To start, 30 data points for each experimental condition can be considered for the study. Depending on the size of the effect, more or fewer data points will be necessary to detect a significant difference between experimental conditions.

Both the input data and the users can be 'reused' in experimental conditions. If the same input items are used across conditions but not the same users, there is a natural pairing for the input items across conditions and the design can be considered a within-subjects design. When the same users participate in multiple conditions but the input items are different, there is a natural pairing of data points based on the users who participate in each condition; this can also be considered a within-subjects design. The researcher should choose one of these approaches and be careful to submit the data in the appropriate manner to the statistics software used.

When an independent variable is treated as a within-subjects variable and subjects participate in multiple conditions, the order of conditions should be randomized per user to avoid bias due to order of conditions. The analysis that is most appropriate depends on the number of variables and conditions. When there is one independent variable with two conditions, a paired samples t-test is the most appropriate analysis. When there are more variables or more than two conditions, a repeated measures ANOVA is most appropriate for the within-subjects independent variables. When there are more than two conditions, post hoc analysis will need to be conducted when a significant effect is found.

When an independent variable is treated as a between-subjects variable, the subjects participate in only one of its conditions. With multiple independent variables, they can all be designed as between-subjects variables and subjects will participate in only one condition of the study. When there is only one variable with two conditions, an independent samples t-test is appropriate. When there are more variables or more conditions, an ANOVA should be conducted. When significant effects are found for variables with more than two conditions, post hoc analysis will be needed to identify which pairs of conditions are statistically different.

Following the same design principle for all variables is the most straightforward approach for conducting the statistical analysis. However, it is possible to combine both within- and between-subjects principles in one study. The analysis has to be adjusted to take this into account so that it is conducted in the correct way and has the most power to discover an effect if it exists.

Applied Example

The developer decides to use a within-subjects design for the study with one independent variable and two conditions. In principle, each user will solve one problem in each condition. However, since it is difficult to recruit a large number of biomedical researchers in a timely manner, it is decided to ask each to solve two problems in each experimental condition. This provides the developer with two data points per user in each condition. As a result, if few users can be recruited, it may still be possible to gather enough data for a statistical analysis.

Since it is a within-subjects design, special care is needed to avoid an ordering effect. The order of the experimental conditions is reversed for half of the users (new algorithm followed by old algorithm versus old algorithm followed by new algorithm) as are the tasks used in each condition (tasks A- B with the old and C -D with the new algorithm versus tasks C-D with the old and A-B with the new algorithm). The order of problems is kept constant in each condition (not: A-B versus B-A). Although keeping this order of tasks constant is not ideal, each study requires trade-offs and the developer reasons that adjusting the order of tasks within each condition would have limited impact but would complicate the design of the study unnecessarily.

Complete IRB Requirements

The studies in this recipe will require IRB review since users are involved. The researchers should start the IRB procedure as soon as possible after making all study design decisions. While IRB may seem unnecessary in comparison to many clinical studies, a study may reveal incompetence or other potentially damaging results to an individual and so care should be taken that the outcome does not negatively affect the participants. Therefore, the study cannot commence until IRB approval has been received.

Since this is an evaluation of algorithms, the researchers would do well to explain this clearly in the IRB application. Few of the IRB members will have experience with studies in computing that focus on evaluating algorithms. By not associating individual participants with their study results, most IRB issues will be alleviated. For studies such as these, no personal identification information is required as long as study subjects fit the inclusion and exclusion criteria. Moreover, even when performance of subjects is poor, this may very well be due to problems with the algorithms.

The usual requirements for IRB approval apply. The study goal and design will need to be explained, together with the data collection and analysis techniques. The researchers will need to explain how confidentiality of data (or even anonymity if studies are conducted online) will be maintained. Many studies in this category will qualify for expedited review. However, it will depend on the specific rules that apply at the researchers' institution(s).

Applied Example

The developer checks the institutional rules and completes the IRB application. The application includes information on where they intend to recruit users to participate, the methods used and the permission to recruit. He decides to collect only basic personal information, such as the number of years of experience and domain expertise. Such information will be helpful if there are outliers in the data. No other personal identification information will be collected. All information will be kept confidential and, by aggregating the data for each participant, data will only be reported by algorithm.

Conduct the Study

Once all decisions have been made and IRB approval has been received, the study can commence. While waiting for IRB approval, it is an excellent time to organize the more practical aspects of the study, such as identifying and reserving the space, and installing and preparing the system if necessary and possible.

Applied Example

While waiting for IRB approval, the developer installs the two algorithms on identical computers. He also spends time installing and testing the accuracy of the software that is used to present the multiple choice questions and record the answers. After receiving IRB approval, biomedical researchers are recruited and those who volunteer to participate are scheduled for sessions. A few quiet rooms were reserved onsite where the users can work on the study problems undisturbed. With multiple computers, several users can be scheduled during the same timeslot, speeding up the execution of the study. Once the study is completed, the data is extracted, evaluated and analyzed.

Recipe 5: Evaluating Standalone Information Systems Using Subjects

Recipe Summary

This recipe demonstrates the evaluation of a complete information system in its natural environment, as is shown in Fig. A.5.1. It is assumed that the main algorithms and the system's interface already have been evaluated and optimized, and this recipe describes a study where the complete system is evaluated. It is compared to another situation, the baseline condition, where no such information system is available. An evaluation of an entire system usually requires working with users and placing the system in the intended environment or at least in a realistically simulated environment. Both within- and between-subjects designs can be used for these evaluations depending on how well different types of bias can be controlled.

Place in the Development Life Cycle

It is essential to test software in its entirety. Ideally, independent evaluations have been conducted so that the developers can be reasonably sure the integrated system will perform as intended. However, even when integrating superior algorithms, the information system's impact or superiority is not guaranteed but needs to be tested. Furthermore, it is unknown how users will interact with it in its natural environment. A user study is therefore necessary.

When evaluating an information system, it is best to allow sufficient time for users to get used to the system. It is often also interesting to collect data over a longer

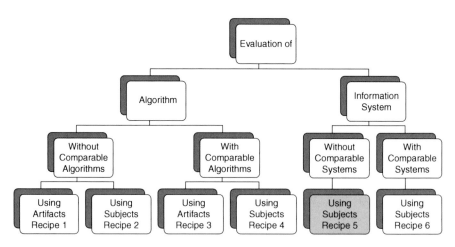

Fig. A.5.1 Standalone information system evaluation using subjects

period of time, after initial training time is completed or at different intervals. With a system evaluation, multiple outcome measures will be of interest. Not all are expected, or required, to show superiority of the new system to make that system valuable. For example, achieving comparable success rates but lower costs for different approaches to therapy may lead to the conclusion that one approach is superior.

The type of study discussed in this recipe is typically a demonstration study of complete systems, i.e., it is a final evaluation, and usually requires a significant amount of time to organize and conduct. A well designed study that shows success of the new system will have significant impact. This will, naturally, affect its success for future use and sales. Such studies often also show how the information system can be expanded or ported to different environments. Unfortunately, the more mature the system is and the more complex it is to integrate it in its natural environment, the more difficult it will become to conduct experiments with random assignments of treatment conditions. In many cases, the baseline data has to be collected before implementation of the study and the evaluation is done with the same group at a later time, which results in a quasi-experiment.

For the current recipe, it is assumed that the information system is intended to be an improvement on a current situation where no such software exists, but where other procedures are in place to solve the problem. This situation is encountered when improvements in software and hardware make novel solutions to existing problems possible where previously no such solutions were feasible.

Applied Example

In this chapter, a fictitious solution to an existing, real problem is used to illustrate the different steps. Clinics where diagnostic tests are conducted often have patients who do not show up for their appointments. When this happens frequently there are negative consequences for both the patients and the clinics. The patients who do not show up get less information and miss their test. As a result, optimal treatment cannot be determined or is delayed. In addition, the appointments are often rescheduled at a later time. This affects the clinic's wait times and expenses. At the time of this problem, the clinic found that following up the appointment scheduling with a well written reminder letter pointing out the importance of the upcoming appointment improved the attendance rate.

It is assumed that an information system could provide a better solution to scheduling patients. The fictitious solution describes an online system that provides educational materials and allows patients to schedule and change their appointment times.[1] When patients are referred to the clinic to schedule a diagnostic imaging test, they can view the clinic calendar online. Using the system, they choose which test needs to be done and then can view the calendar for available slots. Once they have indicated a timeslot, they enter their personal information and they can choose how they would like to be

---

[1] Online systems to schedule appointments developed for the convenience of patients are becoming popular, for example, see http://www.zocdoc.com/.

reminded of their appointment: email, text message, phone call or standard letter. At the end of this process, they are also presented with information on what to expect during the exam, how to prepare and the value of the particular test. Again, they can choose how to read that information: immediately online, by printing or by receiving a copy via email or mail.

Choose the Dataset

The data used as input to the information system should consist of representative input items or tasks. As always, sufficient data points should be available in every experimental condition to allow for statistical analysis. Since an entire information system is discussed in this recipe, the researcher needs to be careful that the study allows for realistic interaction with the information system. Similar to evaluating individual algorithms, data used for development and earlier testing should not be used in the evaluation. Reuse of such data would lead to unrealistic overestimates of the information system.

In general, a study can be conducted that focuses on evaluating the outcome produced by the system or the process of working with the system. When the focus is on evaluating an outcome, the input items can be cases, records or other types of artifacts that require one-time processing by the system. For example, a diagnostic test or a medical record can form the input to the system. The output delivered by the software will be evaluated by the users. In addition, the process itself can be the focus of an information system evaluation. Such evaluation will require a longer interaction between the user and the system. For example, users may be asked to complete a task that requires a series of steps. Each task would count as a data point. The rule of thumb is to get 30 data points per experimental condition. The exact number needed depends on the study design and the size of the effect.

Applied Example

To make an appointment, every patient phones the clinic after receiving a referral from his physician. The input data will consist of patients who agree to participate in the study and who make an appointment using the new or the old system.

Choose the Dependent Variable

When choosing the dependent variable, keep the goal of the information system and the study in mind. This will help pinpoint the relevant and revealing dependent variables. When an entire information system is evaluated in its intended setting, there are usually many dependent variables that are good candidates for inclusion in the study since there are multiple stakeholders interested in a variety of outcomes. However, including too many measurements may be overwhelming to study participants. In addition, the baseline condition for this recipe is a situation without the information system, which will narrow down the choices. Not all dependent variables will be appropriate or practical in both the baseline and experimental conditions.

There often are three groups of stakeholders: the users, the system developers and those requesting the study, such as the buyers (who may be different from the users). Measures should be chosen that are important and relevant to these groups. In addition to considering all stakeholders, it is essential to investigate whether there are outcome measures already being gathered. Such measures may be considered important by different stakeholders. In addition, they may provide good comparison data. Then, there may be measures that have been gathered in the past, for example, during other studies. If possible and if appropriate to the study, include such measures since the stakeholders will be familiar with them.

Similar to other studies that involve users, dependent variables can be categorized as objective and subjective measures. It is essential to maintain a balance and choose enough variables to measure but not so many that the user activities are overwhelmed by measurements. Some objective variables will be important to all stakeholders, while others may be less important to some stakeholders. Most subjective variables, such as ease of use, will be most important to the intended users.

Finally, it is helpful to think of both short and long term interactions with the new system and categorize potential dependent variables in that manner. Some measures will only be relevant for a short term evaluation. For example, the learning curve for a new information system can be measured in the beginning and after a short time. Other measures require a longer interaction period. For example, the average number of cured patients or the rate of correct decisions are typical of such measures.

Applied Example

The developers decide to use a variety of measures. The most important measures are the number of appointments being kept, changed or missed. This is the main interest of the clinic and the clinicians working there. A good evaluation of this system would measure over a sufficiently long period of time, for example, a few weeks (or months) and not just 1 week.

Naturally, the system requires that patients use it and so their opinion of usability and efficiency will also be important, together with their preference for either system. This can be measured with a short survey. The researchers decide to conduct this survey immediately; when the appointment has been scheduled the patient is called and asked the survey questions. This measure cannot be taken when the patient arrives at the clinic since that would lead to missing data for those patients who do not show up.

In addition, there are measures that can be completed automatically, for example, the time patients need to complete making the appointment and the time spent answering the phone with the old system. This can be measured automatically in most cases by logging phone calls and online interactions.

Choose the Independent Variable

As in all studies for the evaluation of an information system, at least one independent variable should focus on the information system and include it as a condition. For this recipe, which describes the evaluation of a new information system which does not have a counterpart, there will be a baseline condition where no information system is used. If other variables are of interest, they can be included as additional independent variables.

When there is no existing information system to compare against, there are still several options for a baseline condition. In many cases, this baseline will be the current state of affairs. For example, a triage process that has been used for years would form the baseline. Comparing to such a baseline would require that users have had sufficient time to be trained and become comfortable with the new system. On the other hand, the baseline may be another new approach to a process or task. If this is the case, both the baseline and the new information system will be new and evaluation could start immediately. For example, when evaluating a new therapy model for teenagers with autism that can be provided in person or online, there is no history of the therapy being used before.

Applied Example

The study will focus on one independent variable with two conditions: the use of the new information system versus the previous approach. The baseline for the imaging clinic is the appointment process as it has been used for years. However, to avoid the situation where some study participants are familiar with the existing process, only new patients will be invited to the study. By applying this exclusion criterion to the study sample, the researchers can ensure that nobody participating in this study will have been trained to use the original system. If patients were included who had been to the clinic several times, they would be familiar with the appointment process and this could affect, either negatively or positively, the way they interact with the system.

Choose the Study Design

When comparing a new system against a baseline without an information system, the researcher should carefully weigh the benefits of choosing a within-subjects or between-subjects design. Practical considerations will impact the choice. The choice of design can help avoid bias, especially when a baseline is chosen that relies on an existing, well known (to the participants) approach. As with all studies, there can be more than one independent variable. Which design principle is followed should be decided for each variable separately. When evaluating with users, the number of data points gathered for each experimental condition will depend on the design and the number of users recruited to participate.

If a within-subjects design is chosen for the independent variable the users will participate in all the conditions of that independent variable. To avoid bias due to the ordering of conditions, the order should be randomized per user so that all possible orderings are included in the study. If more than one independent variable is included that follows the within-subjects design, the user will also participate in all conditions. When there are multiple conditions, it is essential to ensure that the study is not too long so that users will be able to concentrate and perform in each condition. It is also essential that they do not become confused between conditions. Naturally, the order of these conditions should be randomized per user; alternatively, all possible orderings are used and users are randomly assigned to one of the orderings. The analysis to be conducted is a paired samples t-test for experiments with only one independent variable with two conditions. With more conditions or more variables, ANOVA is the appropriate analysis and repeated measures ANOVA should be used for the within-subjects variable. When there are more than two conditions, post hoc analysis will be needed for variables that show a significant effect.

If a between-subjects design is chosen for the independent variable, the users participate in only one condition of the study. They should be randomly assigned to an experimental condition. When there is one independent variable with two conditions, an independent samples t-test is the appropriate analysis. When there are more conditions or more than one variable, an ANOVA is the analysis that should be conducted followed by post hoc comparisons if a significant effect is found. A disadvantage of using a between-subjects design is that the variance within the groups may be higher, resulting in less power to detect an existing effect. However, an advantage of the design is that it helps avoid different types of bias which then may help detect existing effects. Working with more types of users also increases the external validity of the study.

Applied Example

To evaluate the online appointment system, a between-subjects design is chosen. Only new patients are invited to participate to avoid the possibility that some participants have been trained with the existing condition. Each new patient is invited to participate in the study and if the patient agrees to participate, he is randomly assigned to one of two conditions: the normal scheduling method or the online scheduling method. The necessary information is provided for each condition. For the telephone scheduling, the patient is asked to call a different phone number to schedule the appointment. This extra step is included so that both conditions require approximately the same amount of effort to start. Scheduling the phone appointment immediately but not the Internet appointment (patients would need to go online first) would introduce a confounding variable related to the effort that needs to be made to start the appointment process.

Complete IRB Requirements

Once all decisions have been made, the researcher is ready to complete the IRB requirements. As always, the researcher should check with her institution to learn the details of the procedure and the timeline of the review board. No study requiring IRB review can be started without its approval. Most IRB requirements will ask the researcher to specify the study design and analysis procedures. When researchers work with people instead of an existing dataset, additional attention will need to be given to the consent process and the treatment of the personal identification information.

Since the researcher will be interacting with users, the study will not be exempt from review. In addition to deciding on the baseline, study design and analyses to be conducted, the researcher also needs to include the materials to request voluntary consent of the participants and explain how they will maintain data confidentiality. The consent form will need to be clear and easy to understand. The patients' personal identification information should be separated from the study data. In some studies it will not be possible to have participants sign the consent form, for example, when there is no in-person interaction. The researchers should then provide and explain the alternative to the IRB. There are no predefined rules on what is the best way to get informed consent nor does every IRB make the same decisions.

Applied Example

The researchers explain the goal of the study and its design on the IRB form. However, since they are working with patients, they pay special attention to the consent process, confidentiality of data and the assurance that patients will be able to make their appointment regardless of experimental conditions (to maintain the same quality of care).

The researchers create a short explanation that can be delivered verbally and that contains all the necessary information for informed consent. This is included in the IRB information. An assistant will be trained to explain the study to patients and invite them to participate. Upon verbal consent, the patient is assigned a random number. Each such number is associated with one of the two conditions. This random number is associated with the data, not personal identification information. During the consent process, it is explained that participants can always decide not to use the online system and make the appointment by phone. Finally, to ensure that all patients are able to complete their appointment regardless of experimental condition, the process is monitored by another assistant. If the patient is not able to make the appointment in the experimental conditions, he is contacted by an assistant and the appointment is made by phone.

Conduct the Study

After implementing the system, designing the study and completing IRB requirements, the researchers are ready to commence. While waiting for this approval, the researcher can complete many remaining tasks, such as ensuring that the necessary rooms are booked and that all materials are prepared and ready to go. For example, if paper-based surveys will be handed out, it is best to have these packages handy by preparing them in advance. The study can start once IRB approval has been received.

Applied Example

The clinic and researchers have agreed that one nurse will be assigned to the study to direct patients to one of the two experimental conditions. The study will therefore be conducted during her work hours. This nurse has not been involved in scheduling appointments which helps eliminate bias for or against the new system.

When a patient phones to make the initial appointment, he is provided with information about the study and asked to participate. He is informed he can opt out of the study, in which case the appointment will be handled as it was handled in earlier years. When the patient agrees to participate, he is randomly assigned to an experimental condition and also receives a random number that serves as an identification number. When the appointment has been scheduled, the nurse calls the patients and collects the answers to the survey. All collected data are associated with the identification number. When the study is completed, the data is transferred to the researchers for analysis. However, the transferred data does not include personal identification data. The researchers who will analyze the data will not see any personal information but only the randomly generated identification number.

Recipe 6: Comparing Information Systems Using Subjects

Recipe Summary

As shown in Fig. A.6.1, this recipe details how to evaluate an information system and compare it with an existing information system. It is assumed that the systems being compared are complete systems that include various algorithms. The baseline to compare the new system against is another system, often one that is already in place and which the new system should replace if it performs better. Both within- and between-subjects designs can be used for these studies. Because the systems are best evaluated in their intended environment, a system comparison is not an easy task and will take more time than evaluating individual algorithms.

Place in the Development Life Cycle

Once a system has been developed it is essential that it is tested in its entirety. Even when individual algorithms perform as intended, there may be unintended consequences, both good and bad, of using the system in its intended environment. Working with the intended users may also bring new challenges, but often also new ways of using the system, ideas for additional systems or other improvements. This recipe focuses on the comparison between two information systems. The baseline will therefore be another information system.

Similar to the evaluation of a standalone system, comparisons of multiple information systems will include multiple outcomes to be evaluated. Showing superiority for some variables while showing a status quo for others may be sufficient to declare

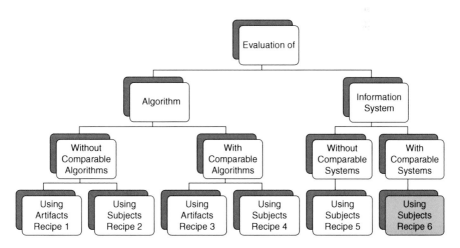

Fig. A.6.1 Information system comparison using subjects

one information system superior to others. For example, Titov et al. [1] compare two versions of Internet-based cognitive behavioral therapy for depression. One version was supported by a technician who provided contact and support but not clinical advice, while the other was supported by a clinician who added clinical advice. Both conditions were compared with another baseline condition which consisted of a delayed treatment control group. The authors found that both online treatment conditions helped patients and did not significantly differ from each other. Since one version was supported by a technician and not a clinician, this version may be cheaper to implement and easier to duplicate. Both conditions also led to improvements not found in the control condition.

A comparison of multiple complete systems is less common than comparing individual algorithms. Comparing two or more systems under similar conditions often is not easy, and there are many potential sources of bias that can influence the outcome. However, an evaluation such as that described in this recipe will often provide a rich assessment by including several different outcome variables. With sufficient control and a set of interesting dependent variables, the study may provide insight into business processes, human interaction with the systems, and ideas or proposals for improvements in treatments, processes and information systems.

This recipe assumes that the information system is compared against an existing information system. This can be a system that has been in place for some time or another system or version of the system that can be put in place in the same manner under the same conditions as for the evaluation.

Applied Example

In this recipe, the fictitious example below is used to illustrate individual steps.

A clinic specializing in diabetics has noticed a disturbing increase in average body weight of the patients they treat. They see this increase in all socioeconomic groups and for all ages. They had some success working with focus groups to encourage patients to lose weight. Unfortunately, they do not have the necessary staff to include all their patients in such focus groups. Therefore, it is decided to try working with online communities. After studying potential solutions and different types of online communities, they decide to compare two types of communities. The first type is a typical online community where participants interact with each other. The second type is a very similar community; however, it has one artificial user. This artificial user is an algorithm that can interact with the community by replying with encouraging comments and making statements containing general advice. The goal of this approach is to ensure that all participants are encouraged, therefore improving weight loss in the group. Online participants will be asked to use the community as a support tool to help each other stick to their diet and exercise regime and also to help each other across hurdles and share practical advice. Participants in the experimental group will be introduced to the artificial user that is the computer program with which they can also interact.

Choose the Dataset

The data used to evaluate and compare the information systems should be realistic. There should be enough data points in each experimental condition to make a statistical analysis possible. It may prove difficult to recruit a sufficient number of users since the more complicated tasks and sophisticated information systems require greater expertise, commitment and a longer time period to complete the study.

Similar to previous recipes, the input to the system or the tasks already used during the development and testing cycles should not be reused during a formal evaluation. Since this recipe focuses on comparing multiple information systems, it should also be pointed out that if an existing system is chosen, this should be used in settings comparable with the new information system. Using default values or a demo version of an existing system would result in a poor study where conclusions about superiority of the new system would be invalid.

Similar to the evaluation of a standalone system, the comparison of two systems can focus on outcomes or processes. When outcomes are the focus, the set of input items are processed by each system and then the outcome is evaluated by the users. For example, decision support systems used to process experiment data would use data input and then suggest a particular action. The focus of the study can also be on a process and how it is supported by the information system. Such evaluations will typically require users to interact for a longer time with an information system.

Applied Example

For the study, data will be collected on weight loss and perceived support in achieving this goal. The data used in the study will also consist of the messages provided by members, their interactions with each other and their interaction with the artificial user in the experimental condition. This data will be collected over a period of time and used to calculate the values on several dependent variables.

Choose the Dependent Variable

There are many possible dependent variables. The study should reflect the goal of the system development; an explicitly stated goal will be helpful in identifying the most appropriate dependent variables. Because comparing multiple information systems in their intended settings can be time consuming, a careful choice of dependent variables is essential. Enough variables need to be included to ensure that conducting the study is worthwhile. However, a balance needs to be maintained because including too many dependent variables will make the tasks less realistic since the measurement activities will overshadow or interfere with the interactions with the systems. This may lower the external validity of the study. Naturally, when dependent variables can be gathered automatically without effort from users and without interfering with their interaction with the system, more information can be gathered.

When entire information systems are evaluated there usually are several different stakeholders in the study. The stakeholders can be thought of as representing three groups: the users, the system developers and a group of stakeholders who may have ordered the study and sometimes may be financially responsible, such as a company that developed a new product. Keeping these stakeholders in mind will help the study designers focus on and balance the dependent variables of interest. Each group will have a specific interest and dependent variables should be included that represent these.

There may be dependent variables that have historically been measured. Such variables are expected to be included in the study. In most cases, these are variables used by stakeholders for ongoing evaluations or for tracking of information for other reasons, such as billing or performance evaluations. There are often also measures that have been gathered in the past and that will be excellent candidates for inclusion in the study. However, care should be taken that these measures are not obsolete. For example, many time-based metrics have become unnecessary with the higher processing speeds of computers. For most users it will not matter whether a question is answered by an expert system in 1.5 or 2.5 s.

When deciding on dependent variables, it is often useful to think in terms of short term measures or long term measures. The first group is related to dependent variables that need to be measured immediately, such as first impressions or a learning curve; while the latter is related to dependent variables that require more time, such as number of errors made over time. In many evaluations, both types will be present. For example, the immediate impact of a system can be measured after each interaction with users, while the long term impact may take days or weeks to become measurable.

Applied Example

To measure the effects of the two types of online communities, three sets of dependent variables are chosen. The first set consists of the main, objective measures that focus on the ultimate goal of the online community participation: weight loss and weight maintenance. Patients who participate will continue to be weighed. This is a measure already in place at the clinic and will be continued for the duration of the study. A second set of objective measures can be collected automatically. These will consist of measures to evaluate the amount of interaction in the community by calculating the average number of posts by a member, the number of responses to posts and the spread of information by calculating the total information in the network and concentration points (hubs of information). Finally, there are also subjective measures included which are collected at the end of the study. They are the perceived usefulness of the online community, perceived usefulness of the advice and information shared online, and the perceived support received from the community.

Choose the Independent Variable

Studies to compare entire information systems will contain at least one independent variable with minimally two conditions: the two information systems being compared. The new system will be compared against an older or other information system. Naturally, as in other studies, additional independent variables can be added to the study if they are of scientific interest.

When designating another information system against which the new information system is compared, it is essential that this new system forms a valid comparison point. It is useless to compare against a demo version of a system or a system using default values if this means the systems are not tuned to deal with the data input or processes. Claiming better performance of a new system would be invalid.

Applied Example

The researchers decide on a simple design with two independent variables. The first is the type of online community: with or without the artificial user. However, to avoid a placebo effect, both conditions include an artificial user and each group is told about that artificial user. In the experimental condition, this artificial user interacts with other users (as intended by the programmers), while in the comparison condition, this artificial user is limited to posting general health messages at predefined intervals. Participants are unaware of the experimental condition to which they are assigned.

The group also has a scientific interest in the usefulness of online communities for patients starting out on their weight loss journey versus those who need to maintain an ongoing diet. It is believed by these researchers that the hurdles to be conquered are different in both groups and that online encouragement is especially useful for weight loss maintenance. The second independent variable focuses therefore on the type of patients: those who are starting out or those who need to maintain a weight loss regime.

Choose the Study Design

When two or more information systems are compared, the design of the study will definitely impact how well different types of bias can be controlled. In comparison to evaluating individual algorithms, it is more difficult to use a within-subjects design where one user would work with different information systems. The time required to learn to use them is typically much longer. If one of the systems has been in use already, this may institute a bias. On the other hand, it is also difficult to place different systems in comparable environments to facilitate between-subjects designs.

If a within-subjects design is chosen for the main independent variable, the different information systems, care should be taken that bias is minimized as much as possible. For example, when users have been working with one of the systems, sufficient training time to work with the new system should be included. When both systems in the study are new, the ordering of the conditions can be varied for the individual users, thus taking away another form of bias. For studies with one independent variable and two conditions, a paired samples t-test is most appropriate, while a repeated measures ANOVA should be used for the designs with more than two variables or more than two conditions. Post hoc analysis is necessary to follow up on significant effects found with ANOVA.

When a between-subjects design is chosen for the main independent variable, the information systems, the study participants participate in only one of the experimental conditions. For each condition, a different group of participants needs to be recruited. Assignment to conditions should be by random selection and each group in a condition should, as a result, be comparable for the characteristics that matter. For example, when age matters, the average age in the different groups should not be statistically different. When there is one independent variable with two conditions, an independent samples t-test is most appropriate, while an ANOVA is most appropriate with more variables or more than two conditions. Post hoc analysis is needed to follow up on significant effects in this case.

When complete systems are compared, the studies become more complex to practically execute and so a mix of variables is often included to answer several questions with one study. As a result, it is more common to have a mixed design where some independent variables follow the within-subjects principle and others the between-subjects principle. The researcher should take care to indicate the correct option when using statistical software packages to achieve the best and most powerful analysis.

Applied Example

The two independent variables in the example study are between-subjects variables. The first independent variable is the online community, and here patients are invited to participate in one of two communities. The second independent variable is the type of patients: patients starting a weight loss regimen or maintaining their weight loss. In this manner, all participants can be recruited at the same time for the study, limiting possible history or learning effects. Patients from each group are invited (random selection from both groups of patients) and randomly assigned to one of the two communities.

Complete IRB Requirements

The researcher should check with his institution for the rules, details and forms to be submitted. The study cannot commence until IRB approval has been received. In studies with complete information systems that focus on patients as users, this IRB process will seldom be expedited since much information is usually gathered that can lead to personal identification and since the continued quality of care cannot be disrupted. With patients, the consent process will need special attention so that any explanation is done at a level that they can understand and quality of care is not affected. Usually studies in medicine include people when they are most vulnerable, and this should be taken into account when designing the study and interacting with these people.

The IRB information will include the goal of the study, a description of the information systems, the study design and analyses to be conducted. The materials used to obtain voluntary consent and the procedure to guarantee confidentiality of personal identification information will need special attention. Ideally, the researcher should avoid collecting personal identification information by working with randomly assigned identifiers instead. Data should be aggregated to avoid people being identified based on their data.

The IRB process will very likely be an interaction between the researchers and the IRB, who are entitled to ask for clarifications and make requirements before allowing a study to commence. Therefore, the researcher should allow sufficient time between starting the process and the anticipated start date of the study. As always, it is helpful to IRB members to have a layman's description of the information systems and their goals, since few members will have much expertise in computing.

Applied Example

From those patients who qualify to participate, a random selection is made and they are then invited to participate. An equal number of participants is recruited for each of the four experimental conditions. Each participant is told how the online community is part of a study to provide better support and encouragement to lose weight and maintain a healthy weight. All participants are informed that an artificial user is present and given the username of that artificial user.

Participants who agree to be in the study can choose their own username and password but are requested to select a username that does not allow for personal identification. Only one nurse in the clinic can map the usernames to actual patients. The researchers collecting the data and conducting the studies will only have access to the chosen usernames. Participants are also told they can quit the experiment at any time without any consequences to their status as a patient in the clinic. At the end of the study, patients will be invited to a debriefing where the study design and results will be shared.

All this information is submitted to the IRB, who require the inclusion of an explanation that clarifies to subjects that the other participants in the online community are also patients and not clinicians. After making the necessary changes and receiving final approval, the study may commence.

Conduct the Study

Once the systems have been completed and tested, the study designed, the IRB requirements completed and all practical aspects taken care of, the study can commence. When a new system is compared with an existing one, it is often best to start with a training period for users so they have time to get used to the new system. Data collection can then start after conclusion of the training period.

With complete information systems, the study often serves as a summative evaluation. It is often beneficial to have a longitudinal study so that impacts that are not immediately noticeable can be witnessed over time. A user study to compare entire systems is complex and time consuming to conduct, but the lessons learned will make it worthwhile.

Applied Example

One nurse at the clinic identifies all patients who would qualify to participate in the study. A random selection is made and the patients are invited to participate. Those who agree choose their username and password and the online community is started. The dependent variables are measured when the online community has been active for 1 month. The researchers collect the data for each user in each community. The subjective measures are collected by the nurses and submitted to the researchers using only the usernames of the patients. The results can then be calculated, analyzed and reported to the scientific community and in patient debriefings.

Reference

1. Titov N, Andrews G, Davies M, McIntyre K, Robinson E, Solley K (2010) Internet treatment for depression: a randomized controlled trial comparing clinician vs. technician assistance. PLoS One 5(6):e10939. doi:10.1371/journal.pone.0010939

Index